Fluids and Electrolytes

T0172440

Fluids and Electrolytes: Essentials for Healthcare Practice is designed to give a solid understanding of fluid and electrolyte physiology and its implications for practice, including acid–base balance and intravenous (IV) therapy, in a concise and easily understandable format.

Chapters incorporate physiological, developmental and practical aspects, highlighting some of the key issues that arise from childhood to old age. This accessible text is presented with clear graphical representations of key processes, numerous tables and contains interesting facts to explore some common myths about human fluid and electrolyte physiology.

A valuable resource for healthcare students, this book also provides a strong comprehensive overview for practitioners, nurses, physiotherapists and paramedics.

Bernie Garrett is a professor at the University of British Columbia, School of Nursing. He worked as a renal clinician for 15 years before becoming a nurse educator. He holds a PhD in information science, specializing in education, multimedia and artificial intelligence. His work is underpinned by a passion for science and technology, and frequently writes on these subjects.

Fluids and Electrolytes

Essentials for Healthcare Practice

Bernie Garrett

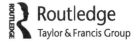
Routledge
Taylor & Francis Group

First published 2017
by Routledge
2 Park Square, Milton Park, Abingdon, Oxon OX14 4RN

and by Routledge
711 Third Avenue, New York, NY 10017

© 2017 Taylor & Francis Group, LLC
Routledge is an imprint of the Taylor & Francis Group, an informa business

The right of Bernie Garrett to be identified as author of this work has been asserted by him/her in accordance with sections 77 and 78 of the Copyright, Designs and Patents Act 1988.

All rights reserved. No part of this book may be reprinted or reproduced or utilised in any form or by any electronic, mechanical, or other means, now known or hereafter invented, including photocopying and recording, or in any information storage or retrieval system, without permission in writing from the publishers.

Trademark notice: Product or corporate names may be trademarks or registered trademarks, and are used only for identification and explanation without intent to infringe.

British Library Cataloguing-in-Publication Data
A catalogue record for this book is available from the British Library

Library of Congress Cataloguing in Publication Data
Names: Garrett, Bernie, author.
Title: Fluids and electrolytes : essentials for healthcare practice / Bernie Garrett.
Description: Abingdon, Oxon ; NewYork, NY : Routledge, 2017. | Includes bibliographical references and index.
Identifiers: LCCN 2016036630| ISBN 9781138197626 (hardback) | ISBN 9781498772433 (pbk.) | ISBN 9781498772495 (ebook)
Subjects: | MESH: Water-Electrolyte Imbalance--nursing | Acid-Base Imbalance--nursing | Water-Electrolyte Balance | Nurses' Instruction
Classification: LCC RC630 | NLM WD 220 | DDC 616.3/9920231--dc23
LC record available at https://lccn.loc.gov/2016036630

ISBN: 978-1-138-19762-6 (hbk)
ISBN: 978-1-4987-7243-3 (pbk)
ISBN: 978-1-4987-7249-5 (ebk)

Typeset in Palatino Light
by Nova Techset Private Limited, Bengaluru & Chennai, India
Printed in Great Britain by Ashford Colour Press Ltd.

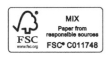

Contents

Contents

Preface

The complex nature of fluid and electrolyte physiology is a subject that often causes anxiety in both the novice and experienced healthcare professional. This book is designed to give the reader a comprehensive overview of fluid and electrolyte function in the body in a concise, accessible, and easily understandable format. It is designed to support professional healthcare students and practitioners in their application of fluid and electrolyte theory to practice. Health professionals such as nurses, paramedics, physiotherapists, physicians, or students in any health discipline may find the content useful. The level of the content is based on an assumption of prior scientific and physiological knowledge, but fundamental aspects are reviewed here briefly to help support those readers who may have less formal education in this area, or for those who have not studied this material for some time.

In this book, I explore fluid and electrolyte physiology in a slightly different format from what is often presented in other textbooks. As healthcare professionals, we are concerned with health, physiology, human behavior, and human growth and development, including the physiological changes that occur across the lifespan. Therefore, I have approached the physiology of fluid balance by incorporating physiological, developmental, and practical aspects here, highlighting some of the key clinical issues that arise from childhood to old age. We will explore how fluids and electrolytes move around the body, how the fluid and electrolyte balance influences other bodily functions, and how disease processes affect fluid and electrolyte physiology, and we will debunk some common myths about human fluid and electrolyte physiology. Initially, we will explore an overview of fluids and electrolytes and then move on to look specifically at the different types of bodily fluids, their functions, and their movement in the human body. We will then explore the nature and functions of the electrolytes in the body and examine the regulatory mechanisms for fluid and electrolyte control. Subsequently, acid/base balance is explored in practical terms, and finally, some of the specific issues associated with the fluid and electrolyte balance through the different stages of human development are examined. In reality, the separation of fluid from electrolyte movement and function in the body is simply a contrivance to help the reader understand their complex functions and interplay, as in the human body these occur concurrently and are very much interdependent.

The text has been designed for use in a variety of different ways: as a textbook, as a reference source, or as a concise guide and primer to the fluid and electrolyte balance for healthcare professionals. The book is laid out for ease of reference and a comprehensive index and a glossary are given at the back. Clear learning outcomes are given for each section, whilst in order to make the subject more interesting for the reader, some related trivia has also been interjected to give context to the material. Specific clinical focus elements are also included, illustrating aspects of particular fluid and electrolyte disorders in order to help the reader to see the application of fluid and electrolyte theory to practical clinical situations. These may also be of use to professional healthcare educators who are covering this material in the classroom.

The book can be used as reference material for those studying this subject at both pre-qualification and post-qualification levels, and as a clinical reference text. It will also prove useful to those studying for specialist practice certification. For more advanced applications, some excellent further sources are cited for those who wish to explore the subject even further.

OVERALL LEARNING OUTCOMES

By the end of this book, you will be able to:

- Identify the functions of fluids and electrolytes in the maintenance of homeostasis
- Explain the roles of fluids in physiological processes in the body
- Demonstrate the roles of sodium, potassium, chloride, calcium, magnesium, and phosphate in physiological processes in the body
- Demonstrate the role of acid/base control in maintaining homeostasis
- Describe the changes in the fluid and electrolyte balance associated with human development and lifespan
- Explain the pathogenesis of common fluid and electrolyte disorders
- Compare and contrast the normal physiology with the altered physiology seen with dysfunction in fluid and electrolyte control
- Relate knowledge of fluid and electrolyte dysfunction to clinical practice
- Apply knowledge concerning normal and abnormal fluid and electrolyte physiology to health issues in your discipline

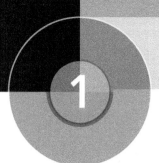

An overview of fluids and electrolytes

SPECIFIC LEARNING OUTCOMES

By the end of this section, you will be able to:

- Describe the function of fluids and electrolytes in the body
- Discuss the functional components of fluids and electrolytes
- Describe the SI units used in the measurement of concentrations and volumes of fluids and electrolytes in the body
- Differentiate the major intracellular and extracellular electrolytes
- Discuss the overall regulation and control of fluid and electrolyte balance

OVERVIEW OF FLUIDS AND ELECTROLYTES IN THE BODY

Disorders of the fluid and electrolyte balance account for a range of serious problems experienced across the lifespan. Bodily fluids, although essential for life, are often regarded with varying levels of repugnance in society, and are frequently considered unclean. This perception is not unreasonable, particularly from a healthcare perspective, as these fluids have often been the vectors for the transmission of infectious diseases. However, this is more of a cultural meme rather than a scientific principle, and in fact, some fluids (such as urine in the bladder) are normally sterile within the body. In early philosophy, water was considered one of the archetypal Greek classical elements, along with air, fire, earth, and aether.[1] Early medicine often concerned practices that involved exploration of the role of the bodily "humors" in an individual's health status, and the therapeutic practices that released them.[2] Bloodletting was an early example of such a practice, and actually persisted well into the nineteenth century. An incision would be made and blood would be drained from a patient in the belief that this would cure or prevent many illnesses.[3] Bloodletting was practiced for a period of at least 2000 years and, in the ancient world, "bleeding" a patient to health was related to the process of menstruation. For example, in ancient Greece, Hippocrates believed that menstruation functioned to purge women of bad humors. Bloodletting was used to treat asthma, cancer, cholera, coma, convulsions, diabetes, epilepsy, gangrene, gout, herpes, indigestion, jaundice, leprosy, ophthalmia, plague, pneumonia, scurvy, smallpox, stroke, tetanus, tuberculosis, and other diseases (even insanity!). Today, our understanding of body fluids and electrolytes is far more sophisticated and, as we shall see, the complex interplay between fluid and electrolyte status and health is better understood. However, we should also acknowledge that much of the complexity of electrolyte and fluid movement around the body remains to be fully explained.

FUNCTIONAL COMPONENTS IN FLUID AND ELECTROLYTE BALANCE

FLUIDS

Technically, fluids are substances, such as liquids or gases, that are capable of flowing and changing their shape at a steady rate when acted upon by a force. For our purposes, we are defining fluids as liquids here. Fluids account for 50%–60%[4,5] of the body weight in an adult and are mainly composed of water with various substances in solution. For physiological purposes, fluids are described as being distributed in two main body spaces: the intracellular fluid and extracellular fluid compartments. These two compartments must have the same osmotic concentrations of fluids within them in order for fluids to remain balanced between them. In addition, fluid in the extracellular space may also be sub-divided into that which is present in the vessels (intravascular fluid) and that which is present in the tissues (interstitial fluid). It is worth noting that fluid transport is a passive process that results in the movement of fluid by osmosis along osmotic gradients established by electrolytes and semi-permeable cell membranes (see below for details of osmosis). Cells cannot actively transport water.

ELECTROLYTES

An electrolyte is a substance that separates in solution into its ionic components and is capable of conducting electricity.[6] These molecules have an electric charge: cations are ions (or groups of ions) having a positive charge and they move towards a negatively charged electrode in electrolysis (chemical decomposition produced by passing an electric current through a liquid). Anions migrate towards the negative pole in electrolysis. In the body, these charges generally balance out within the intracellular and extracellular fluid compartments (see Table 1.1). Electrolytes may be transported around the body by active or passive processes. Passively, electrolytes in solution may be transported by diffusion or carried along as solutes in fluid flow (solvent, or sometimes referred to as solvent drag).

The movement of electrolytes through semi-permeable membranes, such as cell walls, depends on several factors, including the cell

Table 1.1 Relative concentrations of major electrolytes in the body

Intracellular fluid		Extracellular fluid	
Cations		**Cations**	
Potassium	150 mEq/L	Sodium	145 mEq/L
Magnesium	40 mEq/L	Calcium	5 mEq/L
Sodium	10 mEq/L	Potassium	4 mEq/L
Total:	200 mEq/L	Magnesium	2 mEq/L
		Total:	156 mEq/L
Anions		**Anions**	
Phosphate	140 mEq/L	Chloride	108 mEq/L
Protein[a]	48 mEq/L	Bicarbonate	26 mEq/L
Bicarbonate	8 mEq/L	Protein[a]	12 mEq/L
Chloride	4 mEq/L	Organic acids	5 mEq/L
Total:	200 mEq/L	Phosphate	4 mEq/L
		Sulfate	1 mEq/L
		Total:	156 mEq/L

Note: Approximate mEq values are used here for ease of comparison, and please note that "normal" values may vary slightly with different laboratory standards.

[a] Proteins are included as they also have an electrolytic charge.

membrane pore size, the size of the electrolyte molecules (molecular weight), the molecular configuration, and the molecular electric charge. The intracellular and extracellular electrolyte differential is maintained in normal human physiology by both active and passive processes, and key to maintaining this differential is the point at which electrolytes are transported across cell membranes by active processes.

> ### 🌐 TRIVIA
>
> - In an early episode of the 1960s science fiction series *Star Trek*, an unfortunate crewman is reduced to a pile of minerals after an alien dehydrates him. Dr. McCoy, the ships doctor, examines him and states that 90% of the human body is water. This is a gross exaggeration, but has persisted as general knowledge in the public for many years!
> - You can remember the respective charges of anions and cations with the phrase "cations are puss-itive!"

SOME BASIC DEFINITIONS AND SI UNITS

There are a number of terms, definitions, and measurements that are commonly used in describing fluids and electrolytes in the body that are worth getting to know. At a fundamental level, all matter is composed of atoms, which are considered the basic units of matter consisting of a dense central nucleus surrounded by a cloud of negatively charged electrons. A molecule, on the other hand, is an electrically neutral group of at least two atoms held together by chemical bonds. Molecules as components of matter are the building blocks of substances (e.g., H_2O or $NaCl$) and make up our body's fluids and electrolytes.

QUANTITIES AND ELECTRICAL CHARGE

In physiology and medicine, electrolyte quantities in body fluids are usually expressed in Système Internationale (SI) units as a concentration of a specific solute in a given volume of fluid. Measurement units for electrolyte concentrations can be confusing initially, but practically, we are usually interested in *the amount of molecules of a given substance in solution*. It is not very useful to measure substances in solution by grams/liters, as these units do not indicate how many molecules we actually have in our solution. The number of molecules in solution is much more physiologically useful, as it reflects the osmotic potential of the solution in question (see Sections "Osmolarity" and "Osmolality" for a discussion of osmotic potential). Different molecules also have different weights and electrical charges, of course, and we tend to use the measurement of moles/liter as our indicator of quantity in solution (or milliequivalents; see below). Examples of this you will likely encounter include: milligrams per deciliter (mg/dL), milliequivalents per liter (mEq/L), or millimoles per liter (mmol/L). In modern chemistry, the Latin/Greek prefixes uni-/mono-, bi-/di-, ter-/tri-, quadri-/tetra-, and unique-/penta- are used to describe ions in the charge states 1, 2, 3, 4, and 5, respectively.

MOLES AND MILLIMOLES

The mole (symbol = mol) is the unit that is used to measure the amount of molecules (usually expressed as amount in solution; e.g., mol/L). That is, the amount of a substance represented by 6.02×10^{23} atoms, molecules, ions, or elementary units of it. This standard is based upon the measure used to express quantities relative to the number of atoms in 12 g of carbon-12. For example, one mole of carbon-12 weighs 12 g and contains 6.02×10^{23} carbon atoms. Therefore, we can examine other substances relative to this using our molar scale. However, a mole is a large amount of a substance. A millimole (symbol = mmol) is the molecular weight of a substance expressed in milligrams (one-thousandth of a mole), and this is more practically used, as the number of moles is usually very small in physiological measurements. In the USA, the term osmole (osmol) is more commonly used instead of mole (see Section "Osmolarity").

The specific number of molecules of 6.02×10^{23} is known as Avogadro's constant, and is a measure that is named after the nineteenth-century Italian scientist Amedeo Avogadro who, in 1811, proposed that gases are composed of molecules, and these molecules were in turn composed of atoms. He suggested that the different masses of the same volume of different gases could be explained by their respective molecular weights. The actual value of Avogadro's constant was first indicated by Johann Josef Loschmidt in 1865. However, the French physicist Jean Perrin determined an accurate Avogadro's constant by several different methods in 1909, and suggested naming it after Avogadro in respect for his initial ideas.[6]

TRIVIA

October 23 is called Mole Day. It is an informal celebratory day in honor of the mole. The date is derived from Avogadro's constant, which is approximately 6.02×10^{23}. It officially starts at 6:02 A.M. and ends at 6:02 P.M. (but in practice is only celebrated by chemists!).

OSMOLE

The osmole (Osm or osmol) is a non-SI unit of measurement that defines the number of moles of solute that contribute to the osmotic pressure of that solution. A milliosmole (mOsm) is 1/1000 of an osmole. A micro-osmole (μOsm) is 1/1,000,000 of an osmole. It can be confusing as, technically, it is the molecular weight of a solute, in grams, divided by the number of ions or particles into which it dissociates in solution. A 1 mol/L NaCl solution has an osmolarity of 2 osmol/L, as a mole of NaCl dissociates fully in water to yield 2 mol of particles: Na^+ ions and Cl^- ions. Therefore, each mole of NaCl becomes 2 osmol in solution. For example, 9 g of NaCl correspond to 154 mmol of NaCl. The osmolarity of the solution of NaCl, however, is 308 mOsm/L. This difference is due to the number of particles after solvation: one molecule of NaCl in water splits into two ions (Na^+ and Cl^- ions). The term is more commonly used in clinical practice in the USA, and is less popular in Europe.[7]

OSMOLARITY

This is the SI expression of the concentration of osmotically active particles in a solution per liter (volume) of it. It is commonly expressed in mmol/L. Osmolarity is frequently used in clinical practice as we are concerned with osmotic concentrations in particular body fluids. For example, plasma osmolarity = 270–300 mmol/L. Osmolarity is affected by changes in water content, as well as temperature and pressure.

OSMOLALITY

This is also a measure of the concentration of osmotically active particles per kilogram (mass) of the solvent. It is commonly expressed as mmol/kg. Osmolality is usually used in laboratory calculations, or to express the osmotic strength of intravenous fluids. For example, serum osmolality = 282–295 mmol/kg of water. In contrast to osmolarity, osmolality is independent of temperature and pressure. Note that in relatively dilute aqueous solutions (as is often the case in extracellular fluids) there is very little difference between osmolarity and osmolality.

MILLIEQUIVALENTS

The milliequivalent (symbol = mEq) is often used as an alternative to moles in clinical practice, particularly in North America. It is a non-SI measure expressing the electrolytic charge equivalency for a given weight of electrolyte. Electro-neutrality requires that the total number of cations and anions in the body be equal. The technical definition of an equivalent is the amount of substance it takes to combine with 1 mol of hydrogen ions to become electrically neutral. A milliequivalent represents one thousandth (10^{-3}) of a gram equivalent of a chemical element, ion, radical, or compound. When cations and anions combine, they do so according to their ionic charge, not according to their atomic weight. Therefore, 1 mEq of sodium has the same number of charges as 1 mEq of potassium, regardless of molecular weight. For divalent ions such as calcium (Ca^+), the mEq value will be double that of the mmol value. For example, 1 mmol of calcium = 2 mEq.

The number of milliequivalents of an electrolyte in a liter of solution can be derived from the following formula:

$$mEq = mmol / L \times valency \quad or$$

$$mEq = \frac{(mg / 100 \ mL) \times (10 \times valency)}{atomic \ weight}$$

For monovalent electrolytes such as sodium and potassium, the mmol and mEq values are identical. For example, 145 mEq is the same as 145 mmol of sodium.

The number of millimoles of an electrolyte in a liter of solution can be calculated by the formula:

$$mmol / L = \frac{mEq / L}{valency}$$

VALENCY

Valency is another term you will encounter in fluid and electrolyte theory, and occasionally in practice, and it refers to the number of electrons that an atom will lose, add, or share when reacting with other atoms. It is a measure of an atom's combining power with other atoms when it forms chemical compounds or molecules. Technically, it is the maximum number of univalent atoms (originally hydrogen or chlorine atoms) that may combine with an atom of the element under consideration. The concept of valency was developed in the second half of the nineteenth century and was found to be successful in explaining the molecular structures of both organic and inorganic compounds. Many elements have a common valence related to their position in the periodic table. For example, hydrogen has a valency of 1, and so does chlorine, whilst iron has a valency of 3. Valency only describes basic connectivity, and does not describe the geometry of molecular compounds.

HOMEOSTATIC REGULATION AND CONTROL OF THE FLUID AND ELECTROLYTE BALANCE

Homeostasis is the tendency of the body to seek and maintain a balance or equilibrium in its internal environment, even when faced with external changes. An example of this is the body's ability to maintain an internal temperature of approximately 37.2°C when there is a hotter external environmental temperature. Fluid and electrolyte homeostasis is achieved by balancing water and electrolyte intake with losses. Oral intake and absorption in the gastro-intestinal tract provides the main source of fluids and electrolytes, and regulation and excretion occurs at the cellular level and through the kidney and lungs. A summary of daily adult water intake and loss is given in Table 1.2.

The human body controls and monitors its fluid and electrolyte balance, maintaining homeostasis in a number of ways. Two main aspects

Table 1.2 Adult fluid intake and output

Oral intake		Output	
In water	1300 mL	Urine	1500 mL
In food	1000 mL	Feces	150 mL
Metabolic activity		**Insensible loss**	
Oxidation	250 mL	Skin (sweat)	500 mL
Total	2550 mL	Lungs	400 mL
		Total	2550 mL

of fluid balance are regulated: firstly, the volume of fluid outside of the cells in the body; and secondly, the osmolarity of all bodily fluids. Fluid volume in the blood vessels is rigorously controlled by receptors monitoring fluid plasma oncotic concentrations and corresponding neuro-endocrine feedback control mechanisms. This control system is located within the hypothalamus of the brain. For example, thirst is triggered by an increased osmolality of body fluids as identified by osmoreceptors located in the hypothalamus itself. Hypovolemia (low circulating blood volume) also has an important influence on thirst though the renal renin–angiotensin system and arterial baroreceptors in the vasculature (see Chapter 4).

The kidneys also provide primary control over the electrolytes in bodily fluids and, together with the lungs, also regulate the acid/base balance in the body in order to maintain homeostasis. Dysfunction of any of these systems can result in fluid or electrolyte excesses or deficits, and when compensatory mechanisms fail in the body, homeostasis becomes compromised and no longer able to maintain equilibrium with the fluid and electrolyte balance.

✖ CLINICAL FOCUS

Daily fluid and electrolyte maintenance requirements vary among individuals and differing physiological statuses. Intake must equal output, and loss increases with pyrexia, diarrhea, vomiting, gastro-intestinal suction, ventilation, and in polyuria with renal dysfunction. A good rule of thumb is for each 1°C of pyrexia experienced in 24 hours, an extra 10% of fluid is required in order to account for the extra insensible losses. (NB. This does not apply in cases of renal dysfunction.)

Fluids: Their function and movement

2

SPECIFIC LEARNING OUTCOMES

By the end of this section, you will be able to:

- Describe the different physiological fluid compartments in the body
- Compare and contrast intracellular fluid, extracellular fluid and its sub-components, and transcellular fluid
- Outline the typical distribution of fluids throughout the body fluid compartments
- Discuss the regulation, control, and movement of bodily fluids

For physiological usefulness when describing fluid movement and functions in the body, it is convenient to talk of separate bodily fluid compartments (as though they were actual single real entities). In reality, there are many different cellular types with different fluids forming intracellular fluid (ICF), and the nature of extracellular fluid (ECF) in different locations around the body has vastly different characteristics. Nevertheless, categorizing bodily fluids as existing in a few distinctly identified fluid "compartments" is useful for both physiological and medical purposes.

INTRACELLULAR FLUID

ICF (also known as cytosol or the cytoplasmic matrix) is the fluid that is found inside of the cell membrane. In unnucleated human cells (prokaryotes; e.g., erythrocytes), most of the chemical reactions of metabolism take place in this cytosol, whilst in nucleated cells (eukaryotes; e.g., most human cells), many of these chemical reactions take place in the cell organelles. This fluid makes up approximately 70% of a typical cell's volume[8,9] and accounts for the majority (approximately 55%)

of the total body fluid. ICF is high in K^+ and in proteins that are important in the maintenance of osmotic pressure between the ICF and ECF.

Water forms the majority of the cytosol, and concentrations of electrolytes such as sodium (Na^+) and potassium (K^+) are very different in ICF compared to those in ECF. The concentrations of the other ions in cytosol are also different from those in ECF, and the cytosol also contains large amounts of other macromolecules such as proteins and nucleic acids compared with fluid outside of the cell.

Most of the cytosol is water, and pH is maintained at between 7.3 and 7.5, depending on the cell type, whereas the pH of the ECF is maintained more precisely at close to 7.4.[10] Although water is known to be vital for cellular activities, its functions in the cytosol are actually not that well understood.[8,11,12] It is thought that whilst the majority of intracellular water has the same structure as pure water, approximately 5% of it is strongly bound with solutes or macromolecules as the *water of solvation*.[13] This water of solvation (the process by which solvent molecules interact with ions or other molecules) is not active in osmosis and, as it acts as a single entity with the solutes, may also have different solvent properties to pure water.

The majority of cell membranes in the body are freely permeable to water, and water moves between the ECF and ICF simply by osmosis. Water entry into the cell is controlled by osmotically active substances, as well as by ions such as sodium and potassium that pass easily through the cell membrane. Many of the intracellular proteins are electrically negatively charged and attract positively charged ions such as K^+. This partially accounts for the higher concentration of K^+ in the ICF. In addition, Na^+ ions, which are small and have a greater concentration in the ECF, enter the cell easily by diffusion. If this were left unchecked, their entry would continually pull water into the cell by osmosis until it ruptured. The reason this does not occur is because of the active mechanism of the Na^+/K^+ ATPase pump in the cell membrane. This pump mechanism continuously removes three Na^+ ions from the cell for every two K^+ ions that are moved into the cell.[5] The Na^+/K^+ pump is an excellent example of an "active transport" mechanism, since it moves Na^+ and K^+ against their concentration gradients. Energy is required in order to do this, and this energy is supplied by adenosine triphosphate (ATP). An ATP molecule inside the cell is used in the pump mechanism, transferring energy to it. As this energy is used, the ATP is converted into adenosine diphosphate (ADP). See Figure 3.4 for an illustration of the pump mechanism in action. Other ions, such as Ca^{2+} and H^+, are

Table 2.1 Adult fluid distribution by fluid compartment

Fluid compartment	Body fluid (%)	Volume (L)
ICF	55	23
ECF	45	19
Plasma	8	3.5
Interstitial fluid/lymph	19	8
Dense connective tissue/bone water	15.5	6.5
Transcellular	2.5	1
Total	100	42

Note: Values given as approximate examples.[5,8]

exchanged by similar active mechanisms. The result of these processes is that electrolyte concentrations within the ICF are very different from those in the ECF (see Table 2.1).

EXTRACELLULAR FLUID

ECF denotes all body fluid outside of cell membranes. For convenience, it can be divided into two major sub-compartments—blood plasma and interstitial fluid (also known as the third space)—but there are also a number of other sub-categories that physiologists often use in order to further sub-divide ECF.[8] The volume of ECF is typically 19 L, of which 8 L is interstitial fluid and 3.5 L is blood plasma. The typical breakdown of fluids into the various sub-categories is given in Table 2.1.

ECF provides a medium in which cellular nutrients and electrolytes bathe cells and into which cellular waste products can be excreted. It allows for a solute balance between the outside and the inside of the cell, producing a solute gradient that facilities transportation mechanisms (including diffusion, osmosis, and active transport). The normal glucose concentration of ECF is maintained at approximately 5 mmol/L, and the pH of ECF is very accurately regulated at 7.4. The following sub-categories of ECF are worthy of particular attention.

BLOOD PLASMA

The blood plasma accounts for 3–3.5 L of adult body fluid and is often referred to as intravascular fluid in clinical texts as it is constrained within the vasculature. However, it is worth noting that small electrolytes (such as sodium and potassium) are able to pass freely from the intravascular space into the interstitial fluid through the spaces in the capillary walls. Therefore, there is an almost identical electrolyte composition between fluids in the intravascular space and those in the interstitial fluids. The plasma protein albumin is the main osmotically active solute in the plasma as it is far too large to pass into the interstitial fluid and helps maintain the osmotic pressure within the vessels.[8,12]

INTERSTITIAL FLUID AND LYMPH

Interstitial fluid is by far the major component of ECF and is the fluid solution that bathes and surrounds the cells. It is found in the interstitial spaces (tissue spaces also commonly known as "third spaces"). Interstitial fluid also contains proteoglycans (proteins that are attached to glycans) in an extracellular matrix or gel that helps provide cells that are in connective tissues with anchorage. Approximately 8 L of an adult's body fluids are contained in the interstitial fluid and lymph. Lymph is also considered to be a part of the interstitial fluid as the lymphatic system is an open system that drains interstitial fluid from the capillary bed in tissues. The lymphatic system also returns excess fluid, cellular waste products, and proteins into the circulation and has a negative fluid pressure of approximately −5 mmHg. This is maintained by a muscular pumping action as the lymph ducts contain one way valves, promoting fluid movement in one direction draining back to the venous circulation. Because of the number of living cells it contains, lymph is often described as a fluid tissue.[8,12]

BONE AND DENSE CONNECTIVE TISSUE WATER

The fluid in bones and dense connective tissues is clinically significant because it contains approximately 15% of the total body water. This fluid only moves very slowly and is therefore described as inaccessible water, as it is not easy for the body to use it for its processes. Water in the bones themselves makes up approximately half of this water; the rest is located in the dense connective tissues such as ligaments and tendons. This water is an important element of the musculoskeletal structures, but its volume is very difficult to determine accurately and can only really be assessed in the body through magnetic resonance imaging techniques.[14]

TRANSCELLULAR FLUID

Transcellular fluid (TCF) is the portion of total body fluid contained within epithelial-lined spaces, and makes up approximately 2.5% of the ECF, or accounts for approximately 1 L of fluid in the body. Examples of this fluid include cerebrospinal fluid (CSF), gastro-intestinal tract (GIT) fluids, bile, aqueous humor, synovial fluid, sweat, tears, and urine. These fluids are physiologically important to consider because of the specialized functions they support. For example, changes in the GIT fluids can be clinically very significant, particularly in children and older adults. The electrolyte compositions of the various TCFs are very dissimilar, reflecting their individual functions. The most significant specialist TCFs are described below.

GASTRO-INTESTINAL FLUIDS

GIT fluids vary considerably in composition depending upon their location in the gut. The largest component of secreted fluids is water and ions, which are first secreted and then reabsorbed along the GIT. H^+ and Cl^- are secreted by the parietal cells into the lumen of the stomach, creating acidic conditions with a very low pH of 1. H^+ is pumped into the stomach by exchanging it with K^+. This is an active process requiring ATP as a source of energy. Cl^- then follows the positively charged H^+ through a cell membrane protein channel. Further on, in the duodenum, HCO_3^- secretion occurs in order to neutralize the acid secretions from the stomach. Most of the HCO_3^- comes from pancreatic acinar cells in the form of $NaHCO_3$ in an aqueous solution. This results in high concentrations of both HCO_3^- and Na^+ in the common bile duct, creating an osmotic gradient to which water follows.[15] The ions secreted into the GIT primarily consist of H^+, K^+, Cl^-, HCO_3^- and Na^+. Water follows the movement of these ions (see "The movement of body fluids" section below). The sodium plus potassium concentration in stool usually ranges between 130 and 150 mmol/L, and other cations, such as calcium and magnesium, are present at much lower concentrations. The normal stool has an alkaline pH. The main inorganic stool anions are bicarbonate (approximately 30 mmol/L), chloride (approximately 10–20 mmol/L), and a small amount of phosphate and sulfate.

CLINICAL FOCUS

Diseases affecting the GIT commonly cause fluid and electrolyte disturbances. Similarly, intravenous fluid therapy in the perioperative period can affect gastro-intestinal function and have a bearing on postoperative outcome. Careful management of both fluid composition and volume has been suggested to reduce the morbidity associated with interstitial edema, a frequently observed occurrence with contemporary perioperative fluid regimens.[16]

CEREBROSPINAL FLUID

CSF is produced in the choroid plexuses of the ventricles in the brain from arterial blood.[17] A small amount is also produced by ependymal cells (the cells of the thin epithelial membrane lining the ventricular system of the brain). The total volume of CSF in the adult is approximately 140 mL and CSF is produced at a rate of approximately 0.5 mL per minute or 600–700 mL per day. It is reabsorbed by the arachnoid villi into the venous circulation, and the rate of absorption is dependent upon CSF pressure. CSF acts as a shock absorber that protects the brain and also supports the venous sinuses. CSF plays an important role in maintaining homeostasis and supporting metabolic activity in the central nervous system. As CSF is created from blood plasma, it is largely similar to it, except that CSF is practically protein free compared with plasma and has some differing electrolyte concentrations. CSF contains approximately 0.3% of plasma proteins, or approximately 15–40 mg/dL. There are also differences in the distributions of a number of proteins within the CSF in different locations. Globular proteins and albumin are found in lower concentrations in ventricular CSF compared to lumbar fluid.

CLINICAL FOCUS

The pressure of CSF is often measured in clinical practice using lumbar puncture, and is normally 10–18 cmH_2O (8–15 mmHg or 1.1–2 kPa) for an adult patient lying on their side. Assessment of CSF pressure is a useful diagnostic procedure for neurological infective, inflammatory, and neoplastic diseases, including meningitis.

SYNOVIAL FLUID

Synovial fluid is a transparent serous fluid that is secreted by the synovial membrane and is found in joint cavities, tendon sheaths, and bursae in the body and pleural cavities. It lubricates joints and is very similar to lymph. A joint's synovial membrane produces albumin and hyaluronic acid, which give the synovial fluid its viscosity and slickness. In addition, synovial fluid also delivers nutrients to the cartilage and removes waste from it. When a joint is at rest, the cartilage reabsorbs some of the synovial fluid. Then, when the joint is in use the synovial fluid is squeezed out of the cartilage to improve lubrication of the joint. Consequently, joint use is essential to circulating the synovial fluid throughout the joint.[18]

CLINICAL FOCUS

When cartilage is damaged as in osteoarthritis, the body responds by increasing the production of synovial fluid (sometimes by as much as three-fold) in order to compensate for the diseased joint. The excess fluid can cause the joint to become distended, causing further pain.[19]

ENDOLYMPH AND PERILYMPH

Endolymph is also known as Scarpa's fluid after the Italian anatomist who described it (Antonio Scarpa, 1752–1832). It is the fluid that is contained within the semicircular canals of the ear. The fluid is rich in potassium, and contains very little sodium. It is secreted from the stria vascularis in the middle ear. This specialist fluid has a high positive electrical charge (80–120 mV) and carries electrical currents to the hair cells of the inner ear.[20] Perilymph is an ECF located within the cochlea and has a similar composition to plasma, with the major cation being sodium.

AQUEOUS HUMOR

Aqueous humor is also known as ocular fluid and is the clear, watery fluid that is continually produced inside the eye. Aqueous humor is secreted into the posterior chamber by the ciliary body of the eye, and then drains out of the eye via the trabecular meshwork and eventually into the veins of the orbit. The fluid is produced in order to maintain a fluid pressure of approximately 5 mmHg above atmospheric pressure, maintaining the intraocular pressure and globe shape of the eye and providing nutrition to the avascular eye tissues.[21]

FOLLICULAR AND AMNIOTIC FLUID

Follicular fluid is the fluid in a developing ovarian follicle and is rich in hyaluronic acid, one of the main components of the extracellular matrix. The granulosa cells of the developing follicles produce it. Amniotic fluid is the liquid within the uterus that bathes the developing fetus after the first few weeks of gestation. During most of the pregnancy, the fluid is produced almost entirely by fetal urination, but in the first 16 weeks of gestation, additional sources include the placenta, amniotic membranes, umbilical cord, and fetal skin. It has a number of functions that are essential for normal growth and development.[22] It helps to protect the fetus from trauma to the mother's abdomen, it protects the umbilical cord from compression, it has antibacterial properties that provide some protection from infection, it acts as a reservoir of fluid and nutrients for the fetus, and it provides the necessary fluid, space, and growth factors to permit normal development of the fetal lungs.

SEMINAL VESICLE FLUID AND PROSTATIC FLUID

Seminal vesicle fluid makes up a significant proportion of semen and is secreted by the seminal vesicles. Prostatic fluid is the secretion of the prostate gland and contributes to the formation of the semen by making up the seminal fluid. It has a slightly alkaline pH (pH 7.29) and constitutes approximately 25% of the volume of the semen, together with spermatozoa and seminal vesicle fluid. The alkalinity of prostate fluid neutralizes the acidity of the vaginal tract.

Table 2.1 outlines the typical distributions of fluids throughout these compartments. Total body water also varies with gender and weight. These differences are mainly due to differences in body fat (which contains virtually no water).

THE MOVEMENT OF BODY FLUIDS

Fluid moves between the different compartments of the body through a variety of mechanisms. The exchange of intracellular and interstitial fluid is mainly controlled by osmosis in the presence of the electrolytes sodium and potassium.

OSMOSIS

Osmosis is the movement of water molecules caused by a solute concentration gradient across a semi-permeable membrane.[23] It was first described by the French physiologist Rene Dutrochet (1776–1847) and occurs in the body as cell membranes are permeable to the solvent (water), but impermeable to most solutes, and therefore the water molecules move by diffusion (see following chapter) in an attempt to equalize the concentrations on both sides of the membrane. It is a passive process requiring no energy (see Figure 2.1).

The concentration of an osmotic solution is described as its osmolarity or osmolality, and this can be considered to be the osmotic pressure of a fluid. Adult blood osmolality is normally 285–295 mmol/kg H_2O.[5] Water crosses cell membranes freely between areas of low solute concentration and areas of high solute concentration. Therefore, osmolarity tends to equalize across body fluid compartments, primarily as a result of the movement of water rather than solutes.

Tonicity is the ability of molecules in solution to cause an osmotic driving forces and depends upon the solute molecule's size, shape, and electrolytic charge, which affect how it may pass through a semi-permeable membrane. For example, if a molecule is too large, it will not pass through the semi-permeable membrane. Oncotic pressure (also known as osmotic or colloidal osmotic pressure) is the osmotic pressure exerted by the colloids in a solution. An example of this is the pressure exerted by plasma proteins in the blood.

Proteins, organic compounds that remain in the cells, and solutes that move between the ECF and ICF mainly regulate the ICF volume. The membrane in most cells is freely permeable to water, and water moves between the ECF and ICF fluid as a result of osmosis. Potassium

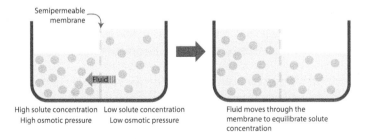

High solute concentration   Low solute concentration
High osmotic pressure   Low osmotic pressure

Fluid moves through the membrane to equilibrate solute concentration

Figure 2.1 Osmosis.

is the major intracellular cation and sodium is the major extracellular cation. Because the osmotic pressure of the interstitial space and the ICF are generally equal, water does not tend to move into or out of the cells. However, changing the concentration of electrolytes on either side of the cell membrane will cause water to move into or out of cells by osmosis. For example, a drop in potassium in the ICF will cause fluid to leave a cell, while a drop in sodium in the ECF will cause fluid to enter the cells.

The endocrine secretions aldosterone, atrial natriuretic peptide (ANP), brain natriuretic peptide (BNP), and anti diuretic hormone (ADH) all act to control the loss of sodium through the kidneys and thereby regulate sodium levels within the body. Aldosterone also acts to regulate potassium levels in the body (see following chapter).[24]

🌐 TRIVIA

What is reverse osmosis? If a force or pressure is applied to a solution with a high solute concentration (also known as the concentrate), the direction of the water flow through a semi-permeable membrane can be reversed. This is known as reverse osmosis and is used in many filtration technologies, including those used in healthcare, such as in the filtration of water for hemodialysis machines.

✖ CLINICAL FOCUS

When body fluids have an osmolarity near 300 mmol/L, they are described as iso-osmotic or isotonic, as their tonicity is approximately equivalent to that of the blood in the intravascular compartment (e.g., 0.9% sodium chloride solution, or normal saline). Hypotonic intravenous (IV) solutions (e.g., 0.45% saline) have a low concentration of electrolytes (a lower osmotic pressure) compared with body cells and can cause cells to swell as a result of osmosis. Hypertonic IV solutions (e.g., 5% glucose in 0.9% saline) have a high concentration of electrolytes (a higher osmotic pressure) compared with body cells and can cause cells to shrink as a result of osmosis. Isotonic solutions (e.g., 0.9% saline) have the same electrolyte concentration (same osmotic pressure) as body cells. If patients require IV replacement fluid therapy, they should have an IV fluid management plan that should include details of the fluid and electrolyte prescription over the next 24 hours and an assessment and monitoring plan.

HYDROSTATIC PRESSURE

Fluid within the body is mostly at a higher-than-atmospheric pressure as a result of a variety of mechanisms (such as being pumped under pressure by the heart or being constrained within a closed compartment under pressure). The pressure exerted or transmitted by the fluid at rest is known as the hydrostatic pressure, and in the human body, fluid generally moves around as a result of this physical pressure exerted upon it. This works together with oncotic pressure to move fluids within the various fluid compartments. The role of hydrostatic and oncotic forces (the so-called Starling forces, after the British physiologist Ernest Starling who first described them in 1896), together with filtration and diffusion, result in the movement of fluid across capillary membranes. These forces are theorized to explain how the movement of water between the vascular and interstitial compartments occurs (see Figure 2.2).

In the capillaries, the blood is described as being under hydrostatic pressure (blood hydrostatic pressure [BHP]) as blood is pumped by the heart and constrained within the vasculature. This tends to force some

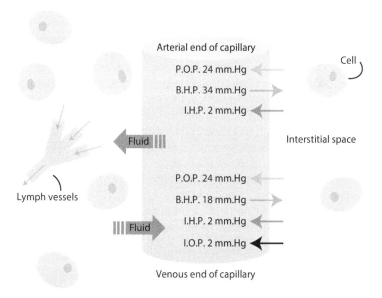

Figure 2.2 Example of the movement of fluid and solutes. BHP: blood hydrostatic pressure; IHP: interstitial hydrostatic pressure; IOP: interstitial oncotic pressure; POP: plasma oncotic pressure.

water through the gaps in the capillary walls into the interstitial space, and as blood flows from the arterial end to the venous end of the capillaries, the BHP at the venous end decreases slightly as a result. The blood also has an oncotic pressure exerted by the proteins and molecules in solution in the plasma (plasma oncotic pressure [POP]), and this acts to pull water back into the capillary, opposing its movement out. The interstitial hydrostatic pressure in the interstitial space exerts a pressure against the flow of water out of the capillaries, and the interstitial fluid also exerts an oncotic pressure (interstitial oncotic pressure) pulling fluid out of the capillaries. Overall, oncotic pressure and hydrostatic pressure must balance in order to oppose net water movement across the capillary wall, and as there is a slight differential in this (with BHP and POP being greater than the opposing forces from the intestinal space), so some fluid remains in the interstitial space. Figure 2.2 illustrates the combination of these four forces that results in only a small excess of fluid remaining in the interstitial space. This excess fluid is drained by the lymphatic system and returned to the venous circulation. The difference between hydrostatic pressure and oncotic pressure is known as filtration pressure, and results in the movement of water and some solutes out of the capillaries.

✖ CLINICAL FOCUS

Tissue edema is the abnormal collection of fluid in the interstitial space. It occurs with increased ECF volume. This may arise in a number of conditions, including heart failure, kidney disease, thyroid disease, liver disease, malnutrition (e.g., kwashiorkor—protein depletion), pregnancy, and as a result of some medications (e.g., corticosteroids or contraceptive pills). If this happens, the interstitial pressure becomes positive due to an expansion of the interstitial compartment with fluid. This may be due to an increase in a solute in the interstitial fluid or an increase in hydrostatic pressure in the venous vasculature. Edema can occur anywhere in the body, but it is most common in the sacrum, feet, and ankles, where fluid collects as a result of gravity. This is known as peripheral (or dependent) edema. Other types of edema include:

- Cerebral edema—affecting the brain
- Pulmonary edema—affecting the lungs
- Macular edema—affecting the eyes

Idiopathic edema is also a term you may encounter that is used to describe cases of edema where a cause cannot be found.

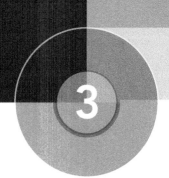

Electrolytes: Their function and movement

3

SPECIFIC LEARNING OUTCOMES

By the end of this section, you will be able to:

- Describe the different major electrolytes in the body
- Compare and contrast the roles of sodium, potassium, chloride, bicarbonate, calcium, magnesium, and phosphates in the body
- Outline the typical distribution of electrolytes throughout the body fluid compartments
- Discuss the regulation, control, and movement of electrolytes in the body

KEY ELECTROLYTES

The electrolytes in Table 3.1 are commonly assessed and monitored in professional healthcare, and they are described in more detail below.

SODIUM

Sodium (Na^+) is a highly reactive element and is the most common cation in the body. It is a relatively small molecule (23 Daltons), so moves fairly easily between fluid compartments and accounts for approximately 60 mEq/kg of body weight. Most of the body's sodium is found in the extracellular fluid (ECF), with a smaller amount sited in the intracellular fluid (ICF) compartment (see Table 1.1). Sodium functions mainly in regulating the ECF volume, accounting for approximately 90% of ECF osmotic activity, and as a current-carrying ion, Na^+ is an essential component in the function of the nervous system. Approximately 40% of the body's sodium is contained in bone, and it is also found within organs and cells. Sodium is important in proper nerve conduction, the passage

Table 3.1 Major electrolyte adult reference ranges in plasma

Sodium	137–145 mmol/L
Potassium	3.5–5 mmol/L
Chloride	96–106 mmol/L
Bicarbonate	22–29 mmol/L
Calcium	2.1–2.6 mmol/L
Phosphate	0.7–1.4 mmol/L
Magnesium	0.7–1.0 mmol/L

of various nutrients into cells, and the maintenance of blood pressure. As a part of the sodium bicarbonate molecule, it is also important in regulating acid/base balance.

Sodium intake is derived from dietary sources and enters the body through the gastro-intestinal tract. The body's need for sodium can be met by a 500 mg/day intake, but dietary intake frequently exceeds the amount required. It is lost through the gastro-intestinal tract and skin, and eliminated by the kidneys. The kidneys efficiently regulate sodium output (see Figure 3.1).

The kidney monitors arterial pressure in the renal juxtaglomerular apparatus and retains sodium when arterial pressure is decreased and eliminates it when arterial pressure is increased through the action of the renin–angiotensin–aldosterone system. This is also regulated by the sympathetic nervous system though a negative feedback system stimulated by osmoreceptors in the hypothalamus and baroreceptors in the carotid sinus and thoracic veins. Other regulators of sodium excretion

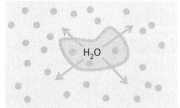

Hyponatremia

H_2O

H_2O

H_2O

Less than 130 mEq/L of Na^+
Water pulled in from ECF and cell swells

E.g. prolonged gastroenteritis resulting in loss of electrolytes, infusing a hypotonic solution

Hypernatremia

H_2O

Greater than 150 mEq/L of Na^+
Water pulled out into ECF and cell shrinks

E.g. prolonged fever, excess sodium in IV therapy

Figure 3.1 Hyponatremia and hypernatremia. ECF: extracellular fluid; IV: intravenous.

are considered to be atrial natriuretic peptide (ANP) and brain natriuretic peptide (BNP). ANP is released from cells in the cardiac atria, whilst BNP is thought to be released by the cells in the cardiac ventricles, although in some animals BNP is released in the brain.[25] The release of both ANP and BNP is stimulated by stretching of the cardiac tissues with increased circulatory volume and also by increased sodium excretion by the kidneys. However, the degree of influence of these hormones in overall sodium regulation remains uncertain.[26,27]

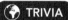

🌐 TRIVIA

Sodium chloride (or common salt) has long been a valuable commodity in human culture. The English term "salary" (as in wages) derives from the term "*salarium*" from the trade of salt. In arid regions, the salt trade has had a strong historical influence in economic development.

✻ CLINICAL FOCUS

- The normal blood sodium level in adults is 137–145 mmol/L.[8,28] In infants, the amount is similar (133–142 mmol/L).[29] Hyponatremia and hypernatremia result mainly from disorders of water metabolism, and the effects of sodium imbalance are usually longer term. However, acute disturbances can also occur. Low sodium levels can result from eating too little salt or excreting too much sodium or water, or by diseases that impair the body's ability to regulate sodium and water. Marathon running can lead to hyponatremia under certain conditions, as sweat contains both sodium and water. Maintaining a low-salt diet for several months or sweating too much during a race on a hot day can make it hard to maintain sufficient sodium levels. Whilst the body can usually compensate and these conditions alone do not normally cause low sodium levels, low sodium can occur in a combination of circumstances. For example, usually only mild hyponatremia occurs in patients taking diuretics. However, patients taking diuretic drugs who follow a low-sodium diet may experience hyponatremia. In some cases, mental illness may cause polydipsia and result in hyponatremia with fluid intake of 20 L a day or more. Moderately low sodium levels may trigger fatigue, confusion, headache, muscle cramps, and nausea, whilst severe hyponatremia can result in seizures and coma.

■ Raised serum sodium levels are unusual, but may occur in diabetes insipidus, if the patient is unable to drink enough water to keep up with urinary loss, and also in unconscious patients who cannot drink in order to keep up with losses. Symptoms of hypernatremia can include confusion, coma, paralysis of the lung muscles, and death.

■ Over the years epidemiological studies have demonstrated that the onset of hypertension is associated with increased long term salt consumption. However, this is not directly associated with hypernatremia, but is thought to be a result of a number of complex physiological changes, including the actions of sodium ions, epithelial sodium channels in the brain activating the renin–angiotensin–aldosterone system, all of which are affected by increased sodium loading.[30]

Tables 3.2 and 3.3 outline the common issues associated with sodium imbalance.[32]

Table 3.2 Hyponatremia

Condition	Clinical causes	Signs and symptoms

The condition where there is insufficient sodium in the ECF (<136 mmol/L in plasma). It is classified as:
 	
1. Euvolemic, where total body water increases, but the body's sodium content stays the same
2. Hypervolemic, where both sodium and water content in the body increase, but the water gain is greater
3. Hypovolemic, where water and sodium are both lost from the body, but the sodium loss is greater
	Burns congestive heart failure, diarrhea, diuretic medications that increase urine output, kidney diseases, liver cirrhosis, syndrome of inappropriate ADH secretion, sweating, emesis	• Central nervous system impairment:
		  • Confusion
		  • Coma
		  • Convulsions
		  • Fatigue
		  • Hallucinations
		  • Headache
		  • Irritability
		  • Lowered consciousness
		• Loss of appetite
		• Muscle spasms or cramps
		• Muscle weakness
		• Nausea
		• Restlessness
		• Vomiting

Table 3.3 Hypernatremia (References 5, 27, and 31)

Condition	Clinical causes	Signs and symptoms

The condition where there is excess sodium in the ECF (>145 mmol/L in plasma, and considered severe hypernatremia at >152 mmol/L). It may be:
 	
1. Hypotonic, where fluid loss occurs without equivalent sodium loss
2. Hypertonic, where sodium intake increases or, more rarely, water moves into cells without equivalent sodium movement (rarely seen in strenuous exercise or electroshock-induced seizure treatment)
	Rare in primary care, but more common in hospital settings where homeostatic mechanisms are impaired or are disrupted: IV therapy, burns, diabetes insipidus, diuretic abuse, excess salt ingestion (more common in children), gastro-intestinal drains or fistulas, hyperglycemic states, iatrogenic, emesis	• Dehydration
		• Dry mouth
		• Abnormal skin turgor
		• Oliguria
		• Tachycardia
		• Orthostatic hypotension
		• Central nervous system impairment:
		  • Lethargy
		  • Weakness
		  • Confusion
		  • Irritability
		  • Myoclonic jerks and seizures
		• Polydipsia
		• Polyuria
		• Thirst

POTASSIUM

Potassium (K^+) is the major cation found in the ICF, and sufficient potassium is essential for normal cellular function. Within the ECF, potassium is not a significant osmotic regulator; however, it plays important roles in normal nervous impulse conduction and in the metabolism of carbohydrates for energy and building amino acids into proteins. Like sodium, potassium also plays an important role in acid/base balance regulation. Potassium is normally ingested from dietary sources and excreted by the kidneys under the control of aldosterone (the same hormone that controls sodium excretion; see Figure 3.2 for a flow diagram of the process). Many foods are rich in potassium, such as tomatoes, bananas, fruit juices, and most snacks and confectionary.

✖ CLINICAL FOCUS

The content of potassium in the ECF in adults and children is approximately 4.5 mmol/L, and the normal blood potassium level is 3.5–5.0 mmol/L.[5,33] In infants, the levels are slightly higher, depending on age (0–30 days: 4.4–7.0 mmol/L; 1–2 months: 4.0–6.2 mmol/L; and 3–11 months: 5.7–5.6 mmol/L).[29] Hypokalemia is defined as a serum potassium level of less than 3.5 mmol/L. Severe hypokalemia results from a level of less than 2.5 mmol/L. It is a potentially life-threatening condition that may result from reduced intake or losses and may even be iatrogenically induced with antibiotic therapy. For every 1 mmol/L decrease in serum potassium, the overall potassium deficit is approximately 200–400 mmol.[34] However, this is a generalization, and individual patients' needs should be assessed carefully. Patients with a mild potassium deficit of 2.5–3.5 mmol/L may only require oral potassium replacement. However, if the potassium level is lower than this, intravenous (IV) potassium should be considered with continuous electrocardiogram (ECG) monitoring and frequent follow-up serum level checks. The serum potassium level may be difficult to replenish if the serum magnesium level is also low, as magnesium plays an important role in the function of the sodium–potassium pump (see "Magnesium" section below).

Hyperkalemia results from a serum potassium concentration above 5.5 mmol/L in adults. As potassium is involved in neurological function, levels higher than 7 mmol/L may result in both hemodynamic and neurologic effects, and levels above 8.5 mmol/L may result in cardiac or respiratory arrest, and may be fatal. However, patients with chronic conditions that cause hyperkalemia (e.g., chronic renal failure) may develop a tolerance to higher serum levels.[35] Management of hyperkalemia is focused on short-term and long-term control. For emergency short-term control, a glucose–insulin IV infusion may be used (which helps transport excess K^+ ions into the cells with the glucose). In patients with hypotension or marked QRS widening, IV bicarbonate, calcium, and insulin given together with 50% dextrose may be appropriate (along with dietary restriction and removal of any potassium-sparing diuretics).[36] Management is in accordance with the patient's signs and symptoms, serum potassium level, and ECG findings. Additionally, in more severe cases, IV calcium may be given in order to alleviate cardiac toxicity (10 mL of a 10% solution over 2–3 minutes). For ongoing management, the aim is to increase potassium excretion from the body.

Renal excretion can be increased by administering IV saline accompanied by a loop diuretic (e.g., furosemide) for patients with normal renal function.[36,37] Gastro-intestinal excretion can be augmented through the use of cation exchange resins such as sodium polystyrene sulfonate or the recently licensed drug patiromer (Veltassa). These both increase fecal potassium excretion by binding with K+ ions in the gut.[38,39] Lastly, emergency dialysis may be implemented for symptomatic patients who are unresponsive to these management measures.

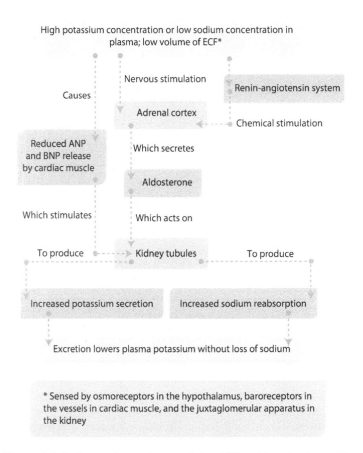

High potassium concentration or low sodium concentration in plasma; low volume of ECF*

Causes

Nervous stimulation

Renin-angiotensin system

Adrenal cortex

Chemical stimulation

Reduced ANP and BNP release by cardiac muscle

Which secretes

Aldosterone

Which stimulates

Which acts on

To produce

Kidney tubules

To produce

Increased potassium secretion

Increased sodium reabsorption

Excretion lowers plasma potassium without loss of sodium

* Sensed by osmoreceptors in the hypothalamus, baroreceptors in the vessels in cardiac muscle, and the juxtaglomerular apparatus in the kidney

Figure 3.2 Sodium and potassium regulation. ANP: atrial natriuretic peptide; BNP: brain natriuretic peptide; ECF: extracellular fluid.

Table 3.4 Hypokalemia

Condition	Clinical causes	Signs and symptoms
Hypokalemia refers to serum or plasma levels of potassium ions below 3.5 mmol/L	Diuretic medications, emesis, starvation and eating disorders (e.g., bulimia), antibiotic therapy (e.g., penicillin), diarrhea, diseases that affect the kidneys' ability to retain potassium (Liddle syndrome, Cushing syndrome, hyperaldosteronism, Bartter syndrome, and Fanconi syndrome), excessive diaphoresis, hypomagnesemia	• Constipation • Fatigue • Muscle weakness, spasm, or damage • Paralysis (which can include the lungs) • Cardiac arrhythmias (an ECG reveals a flattened T wave and more prominent U wave)

Tables 3.4 and 3.5 outline common issues associated with potassium imbalance.

CHLORIDE

Chloride (Cl⁻) is the major anion found in the ECF (see Table 1.1). Chloride plays a role in helping the body maintain a normal balance of fluids, and its movement closely follows that of the cation sodium. Large amounts of chloride are found in both erythrocytes and in the gastric mucosal cells that secrete hydrochloric acid. The body regulates chloride levels by the action of aldosterone, as when sodium reabsorption or loss occurs, chloride follows. The main source of chloride is dietary in the form of sodium chloride, although many vegetables (e.g., tomatoes, lettuce, celery, olives, and seaweed) and grains are also rich in chloride.

Table 3.5 Hyperkalemia (References 5 and 12)

Condition	Clinical causes	Signs and symptoms
Hyperkalemia refers to serum or plasma levels of potassium ions above 5.0 mmol/L	Renal insufficiency, medication (angiotensin converting enzyme (ACE) inhibitors, potassium-sparing diuretics, non-steroidal anti-inflammatory drugs, calcineurin inhibitor immunosuppressants, trimethoprim, pentamidine), excess IV intake, rhabdomyolysis, Addison's disease and adrenal hyperplasia, aldosterone deficiency, Gordon's syndrome	• Fatigue and malaise • Muscle weakness • Cardiac arrhythmias (an ECG reveal a wide QRS complex and a more prominent peaked T wave)

TRIVIA

Seawater has almost the same concentration of chloride ions as human body fluids, but much higher levels of sodium. Hence, drinking seawater is dangerous as it upsets the salinity in the ECF (which increases rapidly), so osmoregulation effects a movement of water from inside cells to outside in an attempt to achieve an isotonic state. So even though you may be dehydrated, if you drink seawater, your cells will actually dehydrate further rather than absorb the water around them!

✕ CLINICAL FOCUS

The human body contains approximately 96–106 mmol/L of chloride in the blood, although children may have slightly higher serum levels at 102–112 mmol/L.[28,29] Imbalances are rare, but hypochloremia may occur with acute diarrhea, prolonged emesis (hypochloremic alkalosis), and sometimes with chronic respiratory disease and acidosis.[12,40] Additionally, hyperchloremia may occur as a result of the use of carbonic anhydrase inhibitors (used to treat glaucoma) and in metabolic acidosis, particularly with severe prolonged diarrhea (e.g., cholera) where fluid and bicarbonate losses accompany anion loss.

BICARBONATE

Bicarbonate (HCO_3^-) is another important anion in the body and acts as a part of the bicarbonate buffer system for maintaining the acid/base balance (pH) in fluids in the body (see Chapter 5). Bicarbonate is ingested from dietary sources (most potassium-rich foods are also rich in bicarbonate, as are baked goods) and is excreted by the kidneys. It is also regenerated by the kidneys depending upon the body's needs (see "Acid/base balance" section in Chapter 5 for more details).

> ### ✖ CLINICAL FOCUS
>
> Normal serum bicarbonate levels are approximately 22–29 mmol/L, although levels are slightly lower in infants and children and vary slightly with age and sex, so local laboratory values should be used for accurate assessment.[5,29] Imbalances are chiefly seen in relation to acidosis and alkalosis, and assessment of the amount of serum bicarbonate can help with determining the nature of an acid/base imbalance in the body and how serious it has become. This subject is dealt with in more detail in Chapter 5.

CALCIUM

Calcium (Ca^{2+}) is a divalent cation that is found mainly in the bone (which contains 99% of the body's calcium). In the ECF, total calcium includes that which is bound with albumin, but the biological effect of calcium is determined by the amount of ionized (separate electrically charged) calcium, rather than the total calcium (see the "Clinical focus" below). Ionized serum calcium is normally in the range of 1.1–1.4 mmol/L (0.045–0.056 g/L) and does not vary with serum albumin levels.[62]

Calcium is one of the most important minerals that the body requires as it is needed for a number of functions, including nervous impulse transmission and regular cardiac rhythm, building strong bones and teeth, blood clotting, and activating digestive enzymes. Calcium also helps maintain the body's acid/base balance. Calcium is ingested from dietary sources (such as dairy products), but unlike the other electrolytes, it is actively transported from the intestinal lining into the bloodstream. Normally, only a small proportion of the calcium that is ingested is absorbed, and vitamin D is required for the active absorption of calcium in the gut. Calcitriol (1,25-dihydroxyvitamin D) is the most active form of vitamin D and is metabolized by the kidneys. It is 100-times more potent than the 25-hydroxyvitamin D that is metabolized by the liver, and promotes calcium absorption from the gut and renal reabsorption, and it enhances bone resorption of calcium.

Free calcium also binds easily with phosphate in the body to form calcium phosphate. There are calcium-sensing receptors in the parathyroid gland, kidney, and other tissues, and calcium levels in the body are tightly controlled by parathyroid hormone (PTH) from the parathyroid glands and calcitonin from the thyroid gland.[41] PTH causes increased osteoclast activity in the bones (thereby releasing calcium), decreases renal excretion of calcium, and promotes absorption of calcium in the gut. Calcitonin acts antagonistically to PTH and lowers serum calcium levels by inhibiting osteoclast activity and bone resorption, and increasing renal excretion of calcium.

✗ CLINICAL FOCUS

HYPOCALCEMIA AND HYPERCALCEMIA

As discussed above, calcium regulation is a complex process that is affected by multiple factors; hence, there are numerous causes of calcium imbalance, and both hypocalcaemia and hypercalcemia are fairly common electrolyte disturbances. Serum total calcium is most commonly assessed and is the measure of non-ionized calcium (bound with albumin, phosphate, and citrate: 53%) and free ionized calcium (47%) in the blood. In adults, total calcium ranges from approximately 2.1 to 2.6 mmol/L, or from 0.09 to 0.105 g/L.[41] In children, the levels vary with age and sex, so local laboratory values should be referred to. The range varies in children and infants (0–11 months: 2.0–2.7 mmol/L; 1–11 years: 2.2–2.5 mmol/L; 12–13 years: 2.2–2.7 mmol/L; and 14–15 years: 9.2–2.65 mmol/L).[29]

However, if serum albumin levels are abnormal (such as in malnutrition), adjustments must be made to the assessment. It is estimated that a 10 g/L decrease in serum albumin is accompanied by a 0.02 mmol/L decrease in total calcium.[42] This may be referred to as "corrected calcium" in laboratory reports. It can be expressed (using the SI units g/L for albumin and mmol/L for Ca^+) as

$$Corrected\ Ca = SerumCa + 0.02$$
$$\times (Normal\ Serum\ Albumin - Patient\ Albumin) \qquad (3.1)$$

For example, if the patient's serum albumin is low at 30 g/L (and we assume a normal serum albumin of 40 g/L), a measured serum calcium of 2 mmol/L should be increased to 2.2 mmol/L using the formula 2 + 0.02 (40–30) = 2.2 mmol/L.

Ionized calcium (that which is not attached to protein) for adults and children is in the range of 1.1–1.35 mmol/L. Ionized calcium is affected by pH, and when alkalosis develops, more calcium becomes bound with protein (see Chapter 4) and the free (ionized) portion decreases, even though the total serum calcium remains unchanged. With acidosis, the opposite occurs, and ionized calcium increases in the blood. These changes in serum calcium are often transient and may not always be symptomatic. However, in order to monitor for acute changes, the assessment of ionized calcium in the blood is desirable for critically ill patients, and may also be ordered from the laboratory in kidney and parathyroid disease. Less than 0.5 mmol/L ionized calcium may produce tetany, and more than 1.75 mmol/L may cause coma.[43]

Tables 3.6 and 3.7 outline the common issues associated with calcium imbalance.

Table 3.6 Hypocalcemia

Condition	Clinical causes	Signs and symptoms
Hypocalcemia is defined as a total serum calcium of <2.2 mmol/L	Vitamin D deficiency, chronic renal failure, parathyroid disease in which excess PTH is secreted, causing more calcium to be absorbed into the bones	• Tetany (muscular spasm) and Trousseau's sign • Paraesthesia and numbness/tingling of hands, feet, and mouth • Seizures • Fatigue • Petechial hemorrhage • Hyperactive tendon reflexes • Cardiac arrhythmias (ECG changes include a prolonged QT segment) • Depression • Osteoporosis (with long-term hypocalcemia)

Table 3.7 Hypercalcemia (Reference 44)

Condition	Clinical causes	Signs and symptoms
Hypercalcemia is defined as an elevated calcium level in the blood (>2.6 mmol/L)	Parathyroid dysfunction, malignancy-mediated hypercalcemia (e.g., tumor parathyroid hormone-related protein [PTHrP] or vitamin D release), lithium or thiazide use, excessive vitamin D ingestion, hyperthyroidism, Paget's disease, Burnett's syndrome, chronic renal failure with secondary hyperparathyroidism, rhabdomyolysis, familial (genetic), idiopathic hypercalcemia of infancy	• Renal calculi • Bone pain • Abdominal pain • Vomiting • Polyuria • Depression • Insomnia • Coma Use the mnemonic: stones, bones, groans, thrones, and psychiatric overtones!

PHOSPHATE

Phosphate (HPO_4^{2-}) exists in the body in both organic and inorganic compounds, and forms approximately 1% of the body weight of humans. The adult human body contains approximately 620 g of phosphorous entirely as phosphate. Phosphate consists of one central phosphorus atom surrounded by four oxygen atoms and is found in all living cells in the body, but like calcium, most (approximately 80%) is found in the calcium phosphate salts in the bone and teeth, where it functions in the formation of hard surfaces. Less than 1% is found in the ECF. The phosphates that are most important to human function are adenosine triphosphate (ATP) and adenosine diphosphate (ADP) for energy, and calcium phosphate for bone mineralization. Phosphate also helps the body to absorb and use calcium, together with magnesium, vitamin D, and vitamin C. It is absorbed in the gut and is abundant in the diet (e.g., in eggs, dairy, wheat, beans, and most processed foods). Intestinal absorption of phosphate is efficient and minimally regulated.[45] The kidney is the major regulator of phosphate, where it is closely linked with calcium metabolism in the body under the influence of vitamin D and PTH. PTH promotes the release of phosphate from the bones (with increased osteoclast activity and associated calcium release), but reduces the reabsorption of phosphate from filtrate in the proximal tubule of the kidney, increasing its overall loss from the body in urine. Other hormones, including thyroid, insulin, glucagon, glucocorticosteroid, and thyrocalcitonin, also play minor roles in the regulation of phosphate metabolism. The kidney filters 90% of the plasma phosphate and reabsorbs it in the tubules as required. In states of hypophosphatemia, the kidney can reabsorb the filtered phosphates very efficiently, reducing the amount excreted in the urine virtually to zero.[46]

Tables 3.8 and 3.9 outline common issues associated with phosphate imbalance.

Table 3.8 Hypophosphatemia

Condition	Clinical causes	Signs and symptoms
A lowered level of phosphate in the blood is known as hypophosphatemia (<0.8 mmol/L)	Hypercalcemia, malnourishment (especially in chronic alcoholism), refeeding following prolonged starvation (refeeding syndrome), respiratory acidosis (see Chapter 5), malabsorption with a lack of vitamin D or the overuse of phosphate-binding antacids	• Muscle dysfunction (cramps and weakness) • Cell membrane failure (due to low ATP) • Cognitive dysfunction (confusion or coma) • Immunosuppression (due to leukocyte dysfunction) • Large pulp chambers in the teeth with prolonged insufficiency

Table 3.9 Hyerphosphatemia (References 47 and 48)

Condition	Clinical causes	Signs and symptoms
A high level of phosphate in the blood is known as hyperphosphatemia (>1.4 mmol/L)	Hyperphosphatemia is rare but may be seen with chronic renal failure as the kidneys fail to excrete phosphate and there is binding and precipitation of the excess phosphate with calcium in the tissues, osteomalacia, rarely as a temporary result of ingesting sodium phosphate solutions in colonoscopy preparation	• Ectopic calcification (deposition of calcium phosphate in tissues) • Pruritus • Hypocalcemia • Osteoporosis (in chronic conditions) • Secondary hyperparathyroidism

✖ CLINICAL FOCUS

HYPOPHOSPHATEMIA AND HYPERPHOSPHATEMIA

The phosphorus blood test measures the amount of phosphate in the blood, and normal adult values are between 0.7 and 1.4 mmol/L. Children and infants generally have higher levels depending on age (0–1 year: 1.6–2.2 mmol/L; 1–4 years: 1.2–2.2 mmol/L; 5–11 years: 1–2 mmol/L; and 12–16 years: 0.8–1.6 mmol/L).[29] Because of the complex control of phosphate homeostasis, various clinical conditions may lead to hypophosphatemia (see below). The clinical signs and symptoms of phosphate depletion are mainly due to falls in intracellular levels of ATP and decreased availability of oxygen to the tissues due to 2,3-diphosphoglyceric acid depletion in erythrocytes. Hyperphosphatemia is less common, as the kidney can excrete high loads of phosphate in overload conditions. However, it can occur in renal failure, hemolysis, tumor lysis syndrome, and rhabdomyolysis.

MAGNESIUM

Magnesium (Mg^{2+}) is another divalent cation and the adult human body contains approximately 25 g of magnesium. Approximately 60% of the body's magnesium is found in the bones. The majority of the rest is found in cells and a small amount in the blood. Overall, magnesium plays an important role in the sodium–potassium pump and in the production of ATP energy in cell mitochondria. It also promotes the regulation of serum calcium, phosphorous, and potassium levels and is crucial to the body's ability to absorb calcium in the gut. It plays a key role in maintaining the integrity of the neuromuscular system and affects neuromuscular functioning in the same manner as calcium. It is therefore important for maintaining a normal cardiac rhythm, and may also play a role in blood pressure regulation. Magnesium is also a cofactor in more than 300 enzyme systems that regulate a wide range of biochemical reactions in the body, including protein synthesis, muscle and nerve function, blood glucose control, and blood pressure regulation.[49] The absorption of magnesium from the gut is regulated by PTH (which increases its uptake), and the kidneys excrete it passively. Food sources of magnesium include leafy green vegetables, wheat bran, and many nuts and beans.

✖ CLINICAL FOCUS

- Even though it is not as prominent a nutrient as some others, magnesium plays an essential role in numerous biochemical processes that take place inside the body, and its clinical significance may be overlooked.[50] Serum magnesium levels are low at between 0.7 and 1.0 mmol/L in adults and similar values in children, as most is found in the ICF. Newborn infants may have slightly lower serum concentrations at 0.5–1.1 mmol/L.[29] Symptomatic magnesium deficiency due to inadequate intake is uncommon as the kidneys limit urinary excretion of this mineral. However, mild magnesium deficiency (hypomagnesia) may be seen due to a lack of dietary intake and can result in loss of appetite, nausea, and tiredness in the early stages, progressing to dizziness, muscle cramps, cardiac arrhythmias, coronary artery spasm, personality changes, and hyperexcitability as deficiency worsens.[49,51] Apart from dietary deficiency, hypomagnesia can also result from excessive vomiting and/or diarrhea, and malabsorption with gastro-intestinal disease (regional enteritis, Crohn's disease, or celiac disease). Alcoholism is another common cause, in which excess excretion of magnesium into the urine, phosphate depletion, vitamin D deficiency, acute alcoholic ketoacidosis, and hyperaldosteronism secondary to liver disease all contribute to magnesium depletion. Type II diabetes mellitus may also cause hypomagnesia, as increased excretion of magnesium in the urine occurs in this disorder.[52]

- Hypomagnesemia is a differentiated form of magnesium depletion in where there is an abnormally low level of magnesium in the blood. It occurs in the later stages of hypomagnesia, and certain substances and some drugs can also deplete serum magnesium levels by binding with it in the blood, such as phylate, oxalate, osmotic diuretics, cisplatin, and cyclosporine.

- Hypermagnesemia is rare as the kidneys are very effective at excreting excess magnesium, but may be seen in renal failure.[49]

PLASMA PROTEINS

Somewhat surprisingly, proteins are also considered to be electrolytes as they have as an electrolytic charge, and therefore have an electrolytic function. Proteins account for 7% of plasma, and this includes albumin, immunoglobulins, and fibrinogen. The most predominant of these proteins in plasma is albumin, which is found at four-fold higher amounts in the blood than in the interstitial fluid. This concentration of albumin in plasma serves an important osmotic function (providing approximately 80% of the plasma oncotic pressure), and albumin accounts for 50% of the plasma protein content. It also transports many substances and binds with calcium in the plasma. Albumin also has a large molecular mass of 67 kDa, which restricts its movement out of the capillaries. However, if we take into account other solutes that contribute to plasma oncotic pressure (osmolality), these also have significant effects. The half-life of albumin is approximately 21 days, with a rate of degradation at approximately 4% per day.[53]

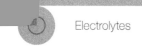

Normal values for serum albumin are 35–55 g/L for children and adults. In infants, the levels may differ with age (0–30 days: 29–55 g/L; 1–3 months: 28–50 g/L; and 4–11 months: 39–51 g/L).[29] When plasma proteins, especially albumin, no longer sustain sufficient colloid osmotic pressure to counterbalance hydrostatic pressure, edema develops. Hypoalbuminemia is a common problem associated with malnutrition and among persons with acute and chronic medical conditions. At hospital admission, 20% of patients are reported to have some degree of hypoalbuminemia.[54,55] Hypoalbuminemia can be caused by various conditions, including nephrotic syndrome, hepatic cirrhosis, heart failure, and malnutrition; however, most cases result from protein depletion in acute and chronic inflammatory responses. Overall, serum albumin is an important prognostic indicator among hospitalized patients, as low serum albumin levels correlate with an increased risk of morbidity and mortality.[55]

THE MOVEMENT OF SOLUTES

PASSIVE DIFFUSION

Diffusion (also called molecular or simple diffusion) is the movement of molecules along a concentration gradient, moving from an area of high concentration to an area of low concentration, resulting in an equal distribution of the molecules by random molecular motion.[6] It is a consequence of the effect of Brownian motion (first described by the Scottish botanist Robert Brown [1773–1858]). In conditions of unvarying temperature and in the absence of external forces, a gradual mixing of material in solution to a state of equal distribution will occur (see Figure 3.3). This is a passive process (also known as passive diffusion), and in this way molecules can pass directly through a cell membrane into the cell, although only small, non-polar molecules (e.g., oxygen) can diffuse easily across the membrane. Passive diffusion is also the main form of transport for materials within cells.

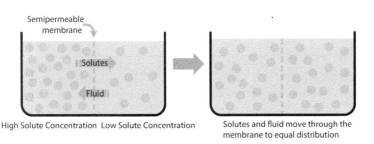

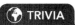

High Solute Concentration Low Solute Concentration

Solutes and fluid move through the membrane to equal distribution

Figure 3.3 Diffusion.

> **TRIVIA**
>
> In 1827, the biologist Robert Brown, looking at pollen grains in water through a microscope, noted that the grains moved in the water, but he was not able to determine the mechanisms that caused them to move. Einstein published a paper in 1905 that finally came up with an explanation.[56] He postulated that molecules of water hitting the tiny pollen grains caused the motion. The pollen grains were visible but the water molecules were not. Brownian motion is one of the simplest of the continuous-time stochastic (random probabilistic) processes.

FACILITATED DIFFUSION

Facilitated diffusion is another form of passive transport, but here the movement of some molecules (such as fatty acids or polar ions, which move less easily) is facilitated by carrier proteins. Larger molecules, especially those that are not soluble in lipids (such as amino acids), do not pass so easily through cell membranes. Likewise, polarized molecules or charged ions (e.g., glucose and sodium and chloride ions) are water soluble, but cannot easily diffuse across cell membranes due to the hydrophobic nature of the cell membrane itself, which repels them. Carrier proteins (also called permeases or transporters) bind to specific molecules and undergo a series of configuration changes that have the effect of carrying the solute to the other side of the cell membrane. The carrier then discharges the solute and reorients in the membrane back to its original state. A specific carrier will transport only a small range of related molecules (see Figure 3.4).[56]

Facilitated diffusion may occur across cell membranes and is similar to simple diffusion in that it does not require the expenditure of metabolic energy (ATP) and transport is along the concentration gradient.[8,12,57]

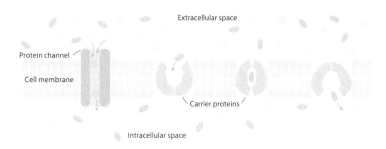

Extracellular space

Protein channel

Cell membrane

Carrier proteins

Intracellular space

Figure 3.4 Facilitated diffusion.

ACTIVE TRANSPORT

Active transport is the movement of a solute against a concentration
gradient using energy (ATP). Passive movement is an effective method
of solute transport for substances to enter a cell because the concentration outside is higher than that inside. However, when equilibrium
is reached and more molecules are required, they need to be pumped
against the concentration gradient. There are many active transport
systems that do this in the human body, and all use a similar biochemical process whereby the molecule outside the cell first binds with a carrier protein. The carrier protein then moves through the cell membrane
assisted by an enzyme and energy from ATP. The molecule and carrier
then separate and the carrier protein returns to its original configuration. It is then available to process another molecule. The following
active mechanisms are well understood in the human body.[58]

1. *The sodium–potassium ATPase pump.* Sodium enters the cell
   by diffusion and is transported out of the cell against an
   electrochemical gradient by an active, energy-dependent process
   known as the sodium–potassium ATPase membrane pump
   (see Figure 3.5). For every two ions of K^+ that enter the cell,
   three molecules of sodium are pumped out. This maintains the
   ICF/ECF concentrations of these electrolytes (see Table 1.1) and is a
   vital mechanism for removing excess Na^+ from the cell.[56,58]
2. *The calcium pump.* This mechanism is vital for muscle contraction.
   It is essential for cells to maintain low concentrations of calcium
   ions for proper cell signaling and contractile functions, and
   therefore body cells employ ion pumps in order to remove Ca^{2+}
   from their ICFs.[59] One mechanism employs a counter-transport
   system that uses a carrier protein (called an antiport) in the cell

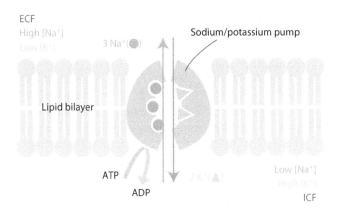

ECF
High [Na⁺]
Low [K⁺]   3 Na⁺(●)   Sodium/potassium pump

Lipid bilayer

ATP   Low [Na⁺]
         ADP   High [K⁺]
                        2 K⁺(▲)   ICF

Figure 3.5 The sodium–potassium ATPase pump. ADP: adenosine diphosphate; ATP: adenosine triphosphate; ICF: intracellular fluid.

membrane to exchange one calcium ion for one sodium ion as the Na⁺ is moved in. This mechanism is known as the sodium–calcium exchanger. The plasma membrane Ca^{2+} ATPase is another carrier protein mechanism that serves to remove calcium from the ICF by active transport.[47,60]

3. *Sodium-linked co-transport.* A sugar or amino acid molecule binds with a sodium carrier protein (called a symport) and is transferred through the cell membrane together with the sodium.

4. *Hydrogen-linked co-transport.* A sugar or amino acid molecule binds with a hydrogen carrier symport and is transferred through the cell membrane together with the hydrogen.[56,61]

FILTRATION

Filtration is the movement of water and solutes from an area of high hydrostatic pressure to an area of low hydrostatic pressure where barriers (such as a cellular membrane) restrict the flow of some molecules. The resulting solution from solutes that pass through a very fine filter (such as a semi-permeable membrane) under pressure is known as an ultrafiltrate. Filtration of solutes may be influenced by molecule size, configuration (shape) of the molecule, and electrolytic charge. For example, glucose molecules are normally too large to be filtered by the glomeruli into the ultrafiltrate in the kidneys, so are not normally found in any quantity in urine.[8,12,47]

SOLVENT DRAG

Solvent drag is also known as bulk flow, and is the movement of both solvent and solutes together. It is a phenomenon that is primarily described in renal physiology, but also occurs in other situations in the body. Solutes are "dragged" along with the flow of fluid. A good analogy is to think of a bath full of water and table tennis balls. If the bath is overfilled, the water will flow over, dragging along some of the balls with it. An example in the body is where solutes in the renal ultrafiltrate are transported back from the renal tubule along with the flow of water, rather than specifically by ion pumps or membrane transport proteins.[62]

✖ CLINICAL FOCUS

INTRAVENOUS FLUID AND ELECTROLYTE REPLACEMENT

Whenever possible, the enteral route should be used for fluid and electrolyte replacement. However, in many cases of acute illness, the only effective solution for rehydration or electrolyte imbalance is to use intravenous (IV) fluids. Various IV fluid and electrolyte solutions are available to the clinician and are broadly categorized into two groups, as described below.

1. *Colloids.* These are solutions of large protein or starch molecules in water that tend to remain in the intravascular compartment for longer than crystalloid solutions. Technically, a colloid solution has particles ranging between 1 and 1000 nanometers in diameter that remain evenly distributed throughout the solution.[5,56] These are also known as colloidal dispersions because the substances remain dispersed and do not settle to the bottom of the container. Examples used in medical fluid volume replacement include Haemaccel, Gelofusine, dextran, hetastarch, or albumin solutions.

2. *Crystalloids.* These are solutions of electrolytes and glucose in water. Crystalloids have additional electrolytes in order to approximate the mineral content of human plasma. The electrolyte molecules readily move across semi-permeable membranes and are the most common IV solutions used in practice. They also have the advantage of being much cheaper than medical colloid solutions. These fluids may be hypertonic or hypotonic, and common examples are given in Tables 3.10 through 3.12. It is worth noting that, normally, fluids with an osmolarity of 600 mmol/L or above should *never* be administered peripherally, and a central venous route should always be used.[5,56,63]

Table 3.10 Commonly used crystalloid infusates for intravenous fluid maintenance

Solution	Indications	Contraindications	Comments
0.9% sodium chloride (Na⁺ 154 mmol/L, Cl⁻ 154 mmol/L)	Rehydration Na⁺ replacement	Hypertension Caution with cardiac or renal failure Edema	Also known as normal saline or n/saline Prolonged use may lead to metabolic acidosis (thought to be due to prolonged bicarbonate-free and high-Cl⁻ solution use) Considered isotonic (osmolality 308 mmol/kg)
0.45% sodium chloride (Na⁺ 77 mmol/L, Cl⁻ 77 mmol/L)	Rehydration Maintenance fluid	As for n/saline	Also known as ½ NS Useful for maintaining daily fluid and electrolyte needs Helps establish renal function Fluid replacement in diabetic patients (as has no glucose) Hypotonic (osmolality 154 mmol/kg)
5% dextrose (D5W) Contains 50 g glucose	Rehydration and is a source of energy	Hyperglycemia Caution with renal failure	Also known as 5% glucose or D5 Used for hydration with no electrolyte imbalance Contains 5 g dextrose Promotes a hypotonic ECF and cellular rehydration as glucose moves into cells Mildly hypotonic (osmolality 252 mmol/kg)

(Continued)

Table 3.10 (Continued) Commonly used crystalloid infusates for intravenous fluid maintenance

Solution	Indications	Contraindications	Comments
4% dextrose and 0.18% NaCl Contains 40 g glucose	Water and sodium depletion and is a source of energy Post-operative maintenance	As for n/saline	Also known as 4% and a fifth glucose saline Dextrose promotes cell rehydration and saline promotes ECF hydration Considered isotonic (osmolality 271 mmol/kg)
5% dextrose with 0.45% NaCl (D5 ½ NS or D5/0.45 NS) Contains 50 g glucose	Hypertonic fluid replacement Replaces sodium and chloride and is a source of energy Post-operative maintenance	As for n/saline	Also known as glucose ½ saline May cause vein irritation because it is acidic (pH 4.4) Hypertonic (osmolality 406 mmol/kg)
KCl solutions: various concentrations of KCl added to n/saline (e.g., 20 mmol KCl in 1 L n/saline)	Electrolyte (K^+) replacement	Hyperkalemia Renal failure	Usually added in IV fluids maintenance Regimes to supply adequate K^+

Table 3.11 Common crystalloid infusates often used in fluid resuscitation/acidosis

Solution	Indications	Contraindications	Comments
Lactated Ringer's solution (Na^+ 13 mmol/L, Cl^- 109 mmol/L, lactate 28 mmol/L, K^+ 4 mmol/L, Ca^+ 3 mmol/L)	Mimics blood electrolytes Acute dehydration with electrolyte imbalance Burns Acidosis Diabetic coma Post-operative maintenance	Caution in diabetes mellitus as LR may exacerbate lactic acidosis Liver disease Cardiac failure Not a maintenance solution due to high Cl^- content and lactate	Also known as lactated Ringers (LR) solution or Ringer's solution Developed by Dr. Sydney Ringer in the 1880s Has a metabolic alkalinizing effect, as lactate is a precursor of bicarbonate (metabolized to H_2O and CO_2, and reduces free H^+ ions) Considered to be isotonic (osmolality 275 mmol/kg)
Hartmann's solution (Na^+ 131 mmol/L, Cl^- 111 mmol/L, lactate 29 mmol/L, K^+ 5 mmol/L, Ca^+ 4 mmol/L)	As for lactated Ringer's solution	As for lactated Ringer's solution	Also known as compound sodium lactate Developed by Dr. Alexis Hartmann in 1932, who modified Ringer's original solution Frequently used in the UK Otherwise comments as for lactated Ringer's solution
PlasmaLyte A (Na^+ 140 mmol/L, Cl^- 98 mmol/L, acetate 27 mmol/L, K^+ 5 mmol/L, gluconate 23 mmol/L)	As for LR's solution	As for lactated Ringer's solution	Also known as PlasmaLyte A newer fluid that uses acetate instead of lactate Useful in cases of lactate metabolism impairment

Table 3.12 Common colloid infusates (References 63 through 65)

Solution	Indications	Contraindications	Comments
Albumin 25%	Hypovolemic shock	Hypersensitivity	Also known as plasma expanders
Dextran 70	Burns	Hypertension	Should not be infused cold
Gelofusine	Hemorrhage	Congestive heart failure	Do not mix with citrated blood
Haemaccel 3.5%	Septicemia	Pulmonary edema	Most technically hypertonic due to colloid osmotic component (although Gelaspan is isotonic)
Gelaspan	Heart/lung bypass machine priming		Recent evidence suggests colloids may be no more effective than crystalloids for volume replacement

CALCULATING IV FLUID AND ELECTROLYTE REPLACEMENT

The prescription of IV fluids is not an exact science, and generally a physician is required to write orders for IV fluids (although in some countries other practitioners are legally entitled to do so). Local guidelines/policies may also empower other healthcare professionals (such as nurse specialists/practitioners or paramedics) to initiate IV solutions within specific limitations. Initially, the clinician should consider whether the need for IV fluids is for fluid maintenance or fluid resuscitation, as these require very different approaches. The prescription of IV fluids can be made simpler by considering five Rs when planning therapy: **R**esuscitation or **R**outine Maintenance, **R**edistribution (consideration of where it will go once delivered), **R**eplacement (of losses), and frequent **R**eassessment.[63,66]

IV FLUID ROUTINE MAINTENANCE

The purpose here is to replace ongoing losses under normal physiological conditions. IV replacement for fluid maintenance is used when the patient is not expected to eat or drink normally for a prolonged period of time. In general, patients who are afebrile, not eating, or not physically active require less than 1 L of free water daily. Patients with renal or edematous states (e.g., cirrhosis, renal failure, or heart failure) require far lower quantities of maintenance fluids (as their fluid output is compromised) and a senior physician should always be consulted before initiating therapy. An initial question to be asked before starting any IV maintenance therapy is: "Is this patient's renal function normal?" Likewise, in the case of infants and children, a pediatrician should always be consulted before starting an IV maintenance regime.

It is worth noting that the normal daily volumes given in Table 1.2 are *minimum* requirements. There are three approaches that are generally used by clinicians in order to establish the appropriate daily fluid volume for IV fluid maintenance in practice:

1. Calculate volume maintenance based on the average adult requirement of 30–40 mL/kg/day (e.g., 35 mL/kg/day)
2. Use the "4/2/1" rule of thumb:
   a. 4 mL/kg/hour for the first 10 kg (0–10 kg)
   b. 2 mL/kg/hour for the next 10 kg (11–20 kg)
   c. 1 mL/kg/hour for remaining weight (21 kg and up)
3. Use the weight in kg + 40 = mL/hour rule of thumb

All of these approaches will give similar results, although the first is simple to implement and recommended.[63,64] For example, for an 80 kg euvolemic adult man with normal renal function, Method 1 gives 2800 mL/day, while Methods 2 and 3 both give 2880 mL/day. IV fluid volumes are normally calculated to be given over three 8 hour periods each day for convenience.

Once the fluid volume requirement has been calculated, the clinician must next decide on the appropriate regime of IV fluids to be used. Basic daily electrolyte requirements for an adult are as follows[63]:

To replace daily losses and meet the body's needs, the average adult needs a minimum of:

- Approximately 1 mmol/kg/day of potassium, sodium, and chloride.

- Approximately 50–100 g/day of glucose to limit muscle catabolism with starvation.
  - NB. Although this is theorized to prevent starvation ketosis, this will not meet the patient's nutritional needs. For example, adults also need approximately 46–56 g/day of protein, 2000–2800 kcal/day (depending on sex/weight), 1 mmol/kg/day of bicarbonate, and other essential vitamins and minerals.[64]

Given these needs, it is worth noting that a normal saline (NS) IV infusion provides approximately 154 mmol/L of sodium and chloride. This is why NS should not be used continuously as a maintenance fluid in patients with normal renal function, as there is a risk of inducing hyperchloremic metabolic acidosis.[94] The osmolarity of NaCl in blood is approximately 290 mOsm/L, and when selecting IV fluids, it is important to understand the differences between the types of fluid we administer, the osmolality of each solution (see Tables 3.10 and 3.11), and how fluid redistribution will occur. It is also important to recognize that although a dextrose 5% in water (D5W) solution appears isotonic, the dextrose is quickly metabolized in the body and therefore it becomes a hypotonic solution rather rapidly once administered, promoting cellular rehydration and fluid movement out of the ECF compartment. Table 3.13 outlines the respective electrolyte contents of common IV fluids.

Given the electrolyte requirements expressed above, we can assume our 80 kg patient needs a minimum of 80 mmol/kg/day of sodium, potassium, and chloride, and 50 g of glucose. Therefore, three 1 L bags in the following regime would meet the patient's minimum requirements:

1. 1 L of ½ NS with 40 mEq KCl/L added, over 8 hours
2. 1 L of ½ NS with 40 mEq KCl/L added, over 8 hours
3. 1 L of D5W over 8 hours

Table 3.13 Respective contents of a range of standard intravenous fluids

	Na$^+$ (mmol/L)	K$^+$ (mmol/L)	Cl$^-$ (mmol/L)	HCO$_3^-$ (mmol/L)	Dextrose (g/L)	mOsm/kg
NS	154	0	154	0	0	308
½ NS	77	0	77	0	0	154
D5W	0	0	0	0	50	252
D5 ½ NS	77	0	77	0	50	406
Hartmann's[a]	131	5	111	28[b]	0	274

[a] Also contains Ca^{2+} 2 mmol/L.
[b] Metabolized from lactate content.

Table 3.14 summarizes the process for calculating IV maintenance fluid replacement needs.

Eight hourly 1 L IV regimes are most commonly used for adults with normal renal and cardiac function, as fluid calculations per 24 hours are simple and any fluid or electrolytes in excess to requirements will be lost through urine. Where there are renal or cardiac considerations, an IV regime will often be based upon the previous day's urinary output + 500 mL (to account for insensible loss). Some common mistakes in IV fluid replacement therapy include:

- Underhydration and failing to account for fluid losses (e.g., vomitus and diarrhea)
- Inadequate fluid and electrolyte reassessment and monitoring, particularly failing to monitor serum sodium and giving too much sodium (recurrent normal saline [n/saline] infusions)
- Insufficient potassium administration

Table 3.15 illustrates the calculation of drip rates for common IV fluid replacement regimes using gravity feed IV systems. However, if you need to be very accurate with IV fluid administration, a pump or controller must be used, not a gravity feed system.

IV FLUID RESUSCITATION

Unlike fluid routine replacement therapy, the purpose here is to correct acute abnormalities in volume status or serum electrolytes quickly. The patient is normally hypovolemic as a result of dehydration, blood loss, or sepsis, and requires urgent correction of intravascular depletion. Objective parameters should be used in order to assess the volume deficit, including:

- Blood pressure
- Jugular venous pressure
- Urine sodium concentration
- Urine output
- Pre- and post-deficit body weight

The IV fluids described in Tables 3.11 and 3.12 are generally those that are used for resuscitation, depending on whether the aim is to correct acidosis or rapidly resolve hypovolemia. Colloids are believed to not easily cross the capillary membrane, explaining their extensive use

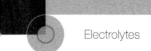

Table 3.14 Fluid replacement prescription (References 12, 27, 63 through 65)

IV fluid prescription requires the assessment of water, sodium, and potassium requirements primarily, followed by consideration of additional calcium, magnesium, phosphate, and chloride requirements. **It is frequently inadequately calculated**, and serum laboratory analysis is necessary in order to monitor the patient's specific needs and responses to treatment. However, the following guidelines based on the pediatric formula (see Chapter 6) work well for calculating general requirements for adults in practice:

Water	35 mL/kg/hour
Sodium, potassium, and chloride	Sodium = 1–2 mmol/kg/day Potassium = 0.5–1 mmol/kg/day Chloride = 1–3 mmol/kg/day (Alternatively, use a 1 mml/kg/day guideline for all)
Consider fluid balance/status	Always review renal function and calculate for other losses (e.g., urine, insensible losses, and wound drainage)

Example: A 70 kg euvolemic man, with normal renal function and no cardiac failure or electrolyte disturbance or abnormal losses who is nil by mouth

Water = 2450 mL/day ≈ 2.5 L/day

Sodium = 70–140 mmol/day

Potassium = 35–70 mmol/day

Chloride = 70–210 mmol/day

A 1 L n/saline IV bag contains: 1 L water, 150 mmol Na^+, and 150 mmol Cl^-

A 1 L D5W IV bag contains: 1 L water and 50 g glucose

A 1 L 4% and a fifth glucose saline IV bag contains: 1 L water, 30 mmol Na^+, 30 mmol Cl^-, and 40 g glucose

30 mmol KCl contains 30 mmol K^+ and 30 mmol Cl^-

So using a regime of 1 bag of n/saline (with 30 mmol KCl added) over 8 hours, followed by 1 bag of D5W (with 30 mmol KCl added) over 8 hours, and then a 1 L bag of D5W over 8 hours, we will meet the patient's daily requirements (giving 3 L H_2O, 150 mmol Na^+, 60 mmol K^+, and 210 mmol Cl^-)

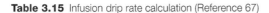

Table 3.15 Infusion drip rate calculation (Reference 67)

To calculate an IV infusion rate, you need to know the following information:

(1) Prescription giving *volume of fluid* to be infused and (2) *time over which it is to be given*

For example, 1 L saline given over 8 hours

If you are using a gravity drip giving set, you will need to know the number of drops in the giving set that make up 1 mL. This is printed on the packaging. Commonly, 20 macrodrops = 1 mL crystalloid and 15 macrodrops = 1 mL colloid

For example, 20 drops of H_2O = 1 mL.

Then simply calculate the following:

1. The number of milliliters to be given per minute
2. Multiply this figure by the number of drops in 1 mL

For example, for 1 L saline delivered over 8 hours:

1. 1000/8 = 125 mL/hour and 125 mL over 60 minutes = 2.08 mL/minute
2. 2.08 mL/minute × 20 drops/mL = 41.6 drops/minute

This is closest to 42 drops per minute, so you would run the infusion at a *42 drops per minute* rate.

in resuscitation. However, a recent Cochrane review of colloids versus crystalloids for fluid resuscitation in critically ill patients found no evidence that colloids reduce the risk of dying compared with crystalloids.[68] Likewise, human albumin has been used extensively for resuscitation, but it is expensive and there is no evidence of its superiority over other colloids or crystalloids.[63]

In cases of severe volume depletion or the initial development of hypovolemic shock where there is no evidence of cardiogenic pulmonary edema, administering 500 mL of an isotonic crystalloid or 0.9% saline rapidly over 15 minutes is recommended, followed by reassessment.[63,66] Hartmann's solution, lactated Ringer's solution, or PlasmaLyte might be used if there is concern for re-expansion acidosis (e.g., in acute pancreatitis). Further fluid boluses up to a total volume of 2000 mL can be given if necessary.[63] In any such case, the assistance of a senior physician should be sought immediately.

In cases of mild hypovolemia, the clinician should estimate all fluid losses (including additional losses through gastro-intestinal disturbances or fever). Then, replacement can proceed at a rate 50–100 mL/ hour greater than estimated losses. Fluid replacement should be on the basis of replacement of the type of fluid lost. Again, the assistance of a senior physician should be sought as soon as possible.

Fluid and electrolyte regulation

4

SPECIFIC LEARNING OUTCOMES

By the end of this section, you will be able to:

- Describe the absorption of fluids and electrolytes from the gut
- Discuss the role of metabolism in creating water in the body
- Discuss the excretion of fluids and electrolytes in the lungs, kidneys, and skin

DIETARY INTAKE

Normally, the body maintains reserves of all electrolytes in order to meet acute needs, and electrolytes are easily replaced without any special dietary requirements. However, with increased sweating (either from activity or heat) or with recurrent vomiting or diarrhea, individuals may lose considerable volumes of sodium and potassium from their body. Usually, these losses can be replaced with dietary intake, but older people and children may be more vulnerable, as they may lose more than they can easily replace through diet alone.[58]

FLUID VOLUME CONTROL

DEHYDRATION

With dehydration, thirst is stimulated by both osmoreceptors in the hypothalamus and kidneys and by osmoreceptors in the heart and vasculature, as well as several negative feedback systems (see Figure 4.1).

Increased ECF osmolarity is sensed by osmoreceptors in the hypothalamus that trigger the brain to stimulate the kidneys (via the renal nervous

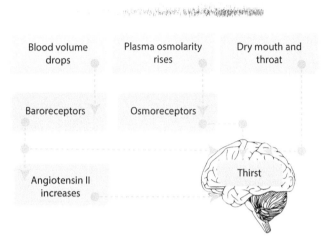

Figure 4.1 Thirst regulation.

plexus) to increase renin secretion. The increased ECF osmolarity is also sensed by the osmoreceptors in the kidneys themselves (in the juxtaglomerular apparatus), and this also triggers the release of renin. Renin acts upon the circulating protein angiotensinogen in the blood, and converts it to angiotensin I. Angiotensin I is then converted to angiotensin II by the angiotensin-converting enzyme found in the pulmonary endothelial cells and in renal endothelial cells (see Figure 4.2). This then has a powerful effect on the production of aldosterone by the adrenal cortex and on the hypothalamus, increasing thirst and stimulating the pituitary to release ADH.[69] This leads to the increased reabsorption of sodium in the kidneys, and water follows by osmosis. In the heart, decreased stretching of the atria and ventricles leads to decreased secretion of atrial natriuretic peptide (ANP) and brain natriuretic peptide (BNP). This also leads to an increase in sodium and water reabsorption by the kidneys. Lastly, the increased osmolality sensed in the hypothalamus and decreased extracellular fluid (ECF) volume sensed by vascular baroreceptors also cause the brain to stimulate the posterior pituitary to secrete more ADH. This causes more water to be reabsorbed from the ultrafiltrate in the kidneys. The net result of these processes is decreased fluid loss and increased thirst.[70] See Figure 4.3 for an overview of these processes.

EXCESS FLUID

With an excess of fluid in the body and a decrease in ECF osmolarity, the same mechanisms lead to increased loss of fluid and decreased

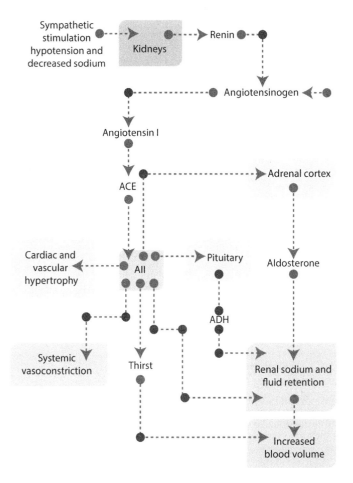

Figure 4.2 The renin–angiotensin mechanism. ACE: angiotensin-converting enzyme; ADH: anti diuretic hormone.

thirst (see Figure 4.4). Decreased ECF osmolarity is sensed by osmo-receptors in the hypothalamus and juxtaglomerular apparatus, causing the kidneys to decrease renin secretion.[70] The renin–angiotensin system's activity is decreased, leading to a decrease in the production of aldosterone in the adrenal glands. This leads to the decreased reabsorption of sodium and water in the kidneys. In the heart, increased stretching of the atria and ventricles leads to an increase in the secretion of ANP and BNP. This also leads to a decrease in sodium and

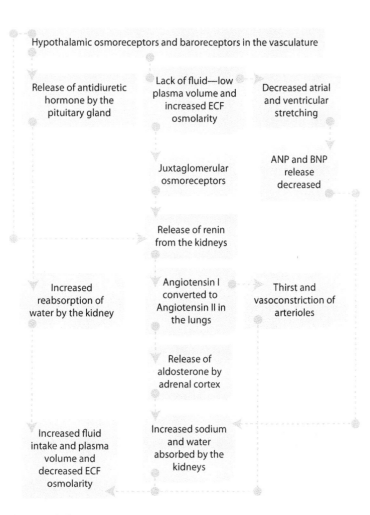

Hypothalamic osmoreceptors and baroreceptors in the vasculature

Release of antidiuretic hormone by the pituitary gland

Lack of fluid—low plasma volume and increased ECF osmolarity

Decreased atrial and ventricular stretching

Juxtaglomerular osmoreceptors

ANP and BNP release decreased

Release of renin from the kidneys

Increased reabsorption of water by the kidney

Angiotensin I converted to Angiotensin II in the lungs

Thirst and vasoconstriction of arterioles

Release of aldosterone by adrenal cortex

Increased fluid intake and plasma volume and decreased ECF osmolarity

Increased sodium and water absorbed by the kidneys

Figure 4.3 Correction of dehydration. ANP: atrial natriuretic peptide; BNP: brain natriuretic peptide; ECF: extracellular fluid.

water reabsorption by the kidneys. Lastly, the decreased osmolarity sensed in the hypothalamus and increased ECF volume sensed by vascular baroreceptors cause the brain to stimulate the posterior pituitary to secrete less ADH. This causes less water to be reabsorbed from the ultrafiltrate in the kidneys.

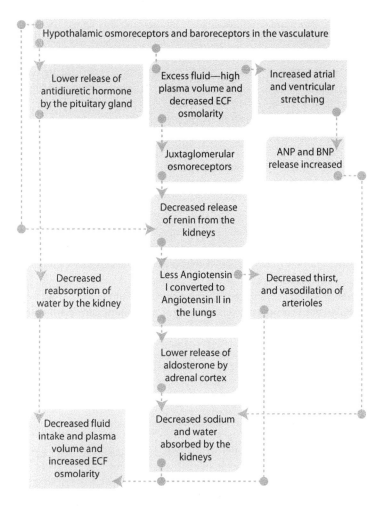

Figure 4.4 Correction of fluid excess. ANP: atrial natriuretic peptide; BNP: brain natriuretic peptide; ECF: extracellular fluid.

ABSORPTION OF FLUID

The small intestine absorbs large quantities of water daily, and this meets the majority of the body's needs. An adult normally consumes 1–2 L of fluid every day, and approximately 6 L of fluid is secreted into the gastro-intestinal tract (GIT) by the salivary glands, stomach, pancreas, liver, and small intestine.[15] By the time this enters the large intestine, most has already been reabsorbed (approximately 80%), and another 10% is reabsorbed in the colon. In the small intestine, where the majority of the absorption of fluids and electrolytes occurs, there is a close coupling between water and solute absorption. In the gut, sodium is absorbed into the cells mainly by the glucose and amino acid co-transport mechanism, such that efficient sodium absorption is dependent on the absorption of these organic solutes.[15] Absorbed sodium is then exported out of the intracellular fluid by the sodium–potassium pump mechanism. This establishes a high osmolarity in the intercellular spaces between the enterocytes, from which sodium diffuses into the capillaries of the villi. Water also follows across in response to the osmotic gradient established by sodium (see Figure 4.5).

If we examine the process of water absorption in the gut as a whole, the transport of water from the lumen frequently occurs against an osmotic gradient. This has been explained by the three-compartment model for the absorption of water,[71] but the exact physiological processes involved remain unclear.[15] Permeability varies across much of the GIT, but it is suggested that the gut epithelium consists of three

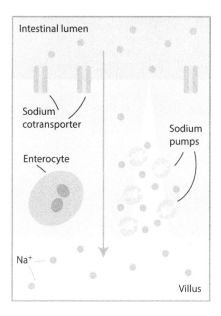

Figure 4.5 Gastro-intestinal absorption of sodium and water.

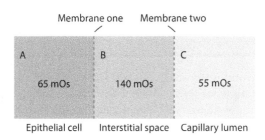

Membrane one   Membrane two

A	B	C
65 mOs	140 mOs	55 mOs

Epithelial cell   Interstitial space   Capillary lumen

Figure 4.6 The three-compartment model for the gastro-intestinal absorption of water.

compartments that are separated by two membranes that differ in permeability (see Figure 4.6).

Water moves against an osmotic gradient from compartment A to compartment C under the following two conditions:

- The osmolarity in compartment B is higher than in compartment A
- The permeability of membrane 1 is lower than membrane 2

The higher osmolarity in compartment B relative to A (and C) provides the driving force for the movement of water from compartment A to B by osmosis. However, as water flows into compartment B, the hydrostatic pressure in that compartment increases rapidly, forcing water to flow through membrane B and into compartment C.

METABOLISM

The metabolism of electrolytes occurs under the influence of a variety of mechanisms, as discussed above. Water is involved in metabolic activities and is actually also created in the body by several processes involving the oxidation of hydrogen in foods (e.g., the catabolism of fat). However, only a small amount of the body's requirements (approximately 300 mL) is actually made by the body each day.[5,56]

EXCRETION

The bodily excretion of water occurs mainly though the kidneys, with some being lost through respiration, perspiration, and a small amount in feces (see Table 1.2). The excretion of electrolytes occurs primarily through the kidneys and perspiration and, like water, a minimal amount is lost through the bowel.[47]

FLUID REGULATION AND SYSTEM ASSOCIATIONS

For convenience in physiology, we view the body as a collection of interacting functional systems, each with its own combination of functions and purposes. Each body system contributes to the homeostasis of other systems and of the entire organism, and each has a role to play in fluid and electrolyte regulation (see Table 4.1).

Table 4.1 Physiological systems and their roles in fluid and electrolyte regulation

Body system	System's fluid and electrolyte functions
Digestive	The digestive system provides nutrients for all of the systems in the body through the processes of chemical and mechanical digestion, breaking down macromolecules in ingested food to basic nutrients that are small enough to be absorbed. Fluid is essential for this process as a solvent, GIT lubricant, and for making up gastro-intestinal secretions. Fluids and electrolytes from dietary intake are absorbed from the GIT.
Reproductive	Conception and the normal development of the embryo and fetus are dependent upon the regular supply of adequate nutrients, including electrolytes. Fluids are essential for the transport of these substances and in the uterus to form amniotic fluid in order to support fetal development.
Immune and lymphatic	Lymph is an essential component in the lymphatic system, and plays an important role in transporting antigens to the lymph ducts, transporting fatty acids around the body, and draining excess fluids from tissues. Humoral immunity requires fluid to transport B-lymphocytes and antibodies around the body.
Muscular	Blood supplies muscle cells with oxygen and nutrients and removes waste products. Essential electrolytes such as calcium are also required for muscle activity.

(Continued)

Table 4.1 (Continued) Physiological systems and their roles in fluid and electrolyte regulation

Body system	System's fluid and electrolyte functions
Skeletal	The bones and teeth require essential electrolytes such as calcium, phosphate, and magnesium to function. Bone water is also essential to the structure of bone. Blood is required in order to transport nutrients to the skeletal tissues and remove waste products.
Nervous	Normal functioning of the nervous system is dependent upon a range of electrolytes, including sodium, calcium, and potassium. The presence of nutrients in blood circulation supports nervous tissue metabolic activity, and this fluid also removes waste products from nerve cells.
Endocrine	Fluids provide the transport medium for hormones throughout the body for moving them from their site of secretion to their site of action. Blood supplies endocrine glands with oxygen and the nutrients from which their various secretions are manufactured, and removes waste products.
Cardiovascular and blood	The circulatory system transports oxygen and absorbed nutrients from the gut to all cells in the body, and removes waste products. Fluid provides the medium for the heart and vasculature to maintain blood pressure and move blood cells around the body. Baroreceptors monitor fluid pressure in the circulatory system. The circulatory system also transports hormones produced by endocrine glands to their target sites.
Respiratory	The respiratory system removes excess water as water vapor during respiration. The oxygen needed for metabolic processes is transported from the lungs in fluid, which also forms the surfactant for lubricating lung tissues. Carbon dioxide—a waste product of cellular metabolism—is transported to the lungs for removal. The acid/base balance is partly regulated through respiratory mechanisms.

(Continued)

Table 4.1 (Continued) Physiological systems and their roles in fluid and electrolyte regulation

Body system	System's fluid and electrolyte functions
Renal/urinary	The kidneys remove excess water from the body and excrete the waste products of metabolism and other toxins as urine. Osmoreceptors in the juxtaglomerular apparatus monitor blood osmolarity. The specialist cells of the digestive system produce metabolic waste.
Integumentary	The skin prevents excess fluid loss from the body and removes water through sweating in order to help regulate temperature. Sodium is also excreted in sweat.

Acid/base balance

SPECIFIC LEARNING OUTCOMES

By the end of this section, you will be able to:

- Describe the roles of acids and bases and pH in the body
- Compare and contrast the regulation of acids and bases in the body
- Outline the three major buffering systems in the body
- Discuss the regulation of the acid/base balance by respiratory control
- Discuss the regulation of the acid/base balance by renal/metabolic control

A vital aspect of fluid regulation in the body is controlling its acidity or alkalinity. In general, we ingest more acidic compounds than alkaline compounds in the body (e.g., amino acids in protein), and produce acids as a byproduct of various metabolic and biochemical processes. Acidity is balanced through buffering in the body and the elimination of excess acids. The body's balance between acidity and alkalinity is referred to as the acid/base balance. Metabolic or respiratory disorders can both result in disturbance of the acid/base balance.[12,56]

ACIDS AND BASES

ACIDS

A substance that liberates hydrogen ions (H^+) in solution is known as an acid. A weak acid only partially dissociates in solution, whilst a strong one dissociates more readily. We also have volatile and fixed acids.

Volatile acids are weak acids that break down easily and can cross the alveolar capillary membrane to be removed in the lungs (e.g., carbonic acid [H_2CO_3]), whereas fixed acids are organic acids that cannot be removed in the lungs, such as hydrochloric acid (HCl).[56]

BASES

A base is a substance that combines with H^+ ions in solution. A weak base only partially combines with H^+ ions, whilst a strong one combines more completely. These may be ingested in our diet or produced by biochemical activity in the body. As bases can accept H^+ ions, they are generally negatively charged substances. One important example is bicarbonate (HCO_3^-), which may be ingested in our diet, but is also regenerated by the kidneys in the body when the need arises.[12,56]

pH

Acidity/alkalinity is measured by the pH negative logarithmic scale that ranges from 0 (strongly acidic) to 14 (strongly alkaline or basic). Negative logs are very small numbers (e.g., 0.000000001), and a negative log is given the expression **p**. Negative logs are used for the calculation of acidity/alkalinity as this is a measure of the concentration of hydrogen ions (H^+) in solution (which is a very small amount). This is therefore known as pH.[56,72]

An acidic solution with a pH of 6 contains 10^{-6} mol/L hydrogen ions (0.000001 mol/L), whereas an alkaline solution with a pH of 8 contains 10^{-8} mol/L hydrogen ions (0.00000001 mol/L; i.e., it has 100-fold fewer H^+ ions in it than the pH 6 solution).

Blood is normally slightly basic, with a pH range of 7.35–7.45. For homeostasis, the body maintains the pH of blood at close to 7.40. The blood's acid/base balance is very precisely controlled (see Figure 5.1), because even a minor deviation will severely affect many vital organs. The body uses several different mechanisms in order to control the blood's acid/base balance.

THE REGULATION OF THE ACID/BASE BALANCE

The regulation of the acid/base balance is broadly controlled by three mechanisms:

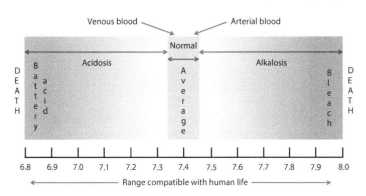

Figure 5.1 pH range in the human body.

1. Buffering—changes in pH are resisted by chemical buffers in the cells and body fluids, which act in pairs almost immediately.
2. Respiratory regulation (in the lungs)—this provides rapid control within minutes of excess carbonic acid.
3. Renal (metabolic) regulation—this is a slow process that takes hours or days to remove H^+ ions and regenerate bicarbonate.

BUFFERING SYSTEMS

Buffer systems provide immediate control by rapidly neutralizing any excesses hydrogen ions. Buffering mechanisms consist of a weak base and a weak acid pair that work together (conjugate) and guard the body against sudden shifts in acidity and alkalinity. There are a number of buffer systems in the body.

The bicarbonate buffer system is the most important of these and uses carbonic acid and bicarbonate, which are readily available in the blood. The normal ratio of carbonic acid to bicarbonate in the blood is 20:1. If excess H^+ ions are present in the blood, then they react with bicarbonate to form carbonic acid. This reaction produces more carbonic acid and less bicarbonate, but the number of H^+ ions in solution remains unchanged. If H^+ ions are removed from the body, such as by vomiting, then more carbonic acid will dissociate into bicarbonate, releasing H^+ ions. The rate of carbonic acid production or breakdown is accelerated in cells by the enzyme carbonic anhydrase.[15]

$$CO_2 + H_2O \overset{\text{Carbonic}}{\underset{\text{Anhydrase}}{\rightleftarrows}} H_2CO_3 \rightleftarrows H^+ + HCO_3^-$$

This system can also help neutralize the effects of strong acids and bases. It helps in the formation of hydrochloric acid within the stomach, where carbonic acid and sodium chloride react to form HCl for breaking down food. A reversal of this process occurs, involving the breaking down of HCl and also the creation of sodium bicarbonate ($NaHCO_3$) in order to neutralize the pH of the chyme leaving the stomach and entering the small intestine. Plasma bicarbonate is primarily regulated by the kidneys and by carbonic acid excretion by the lungs.[12,73]

The phosphate buffer system works in a similar way, but regulates the pH within cells. As the concentration of phosphate is higher in the intracellular fluid (ICF), this buffer system is particularly important within erythrocytes. The phosphate buffer dihydrogen phosphate (HPO_4^{2-}) acts as the weak acid, and hydrogen phosphate (HPO_4^{2-}) acts as the weak conjugate base. When pH decreases as H^+ ions are added, hydrogen phosphate acts as an H^+ acceptor, and when pH increases as H^+ ions are lost, dihydrogen phosphate donates H^+ ions.

$$H_2PO_4^- \rightleftarrows H^+ + HPO_4^{2-}$$

Phosphates are important buffers in the ICF and in the collecting ducts of the kidneys, where they buffer urine.[74]

The protein buffer system is the most abundant buffer system in the body and is of most importance within cells, where proteins are most abundant. The carboxyl group can take up H^+ ions whilst the amine group can liberate H^+ ions.[15]

Intracellular proteins with negative electrolytic charges serve as buffers. They act immediately within cells and at up to 2–4 hours later in plasma. Hemoglobin (Hb) is a key example and makes an excellent intracellular buffer because of its ability to bind with H^+ ions and carbon dioxide (CO_2) to form a weak acid. After oxygen is released in the peripheral tissues, Hb binds with CO_2 and H^+ ions. Hence, venous blood with high CO_2 levels has a lower pH (is more acidic). When Hb binds with CO_2 and H^+, it causes a conformational change in the protein and facilitates the release of oxygen. When the blood reaches the lungs and a highly oxygenated environment, the Hb binds with oxygen, releasing the CO_2 and H^+ ions. The H^+ ions are then buffered by bicarbonate buffers and the resulting H_2CO_3 breaks down to form water (H_2O) and CO_2, which is then excreted during expiration through the lungs.[12,15,73]

RESPIRATORY CONTROL OF THE ACID/BASE BALANCE

Hb blood buffering involves the release of CO_2 from the lungs. CO_2 is mildly acidic, and normal cellular respiration constantly produces CO_2. This would increase acidity as CO_2 and H_2O form H_2CO_3, of which the excess then ionizes into HCO_3^- and H^+ ions. However, the lungs excrete CO_2, and therefore excess H^+ accumulation is prevented. The respiratory center in the medulla of the brain regulates the amount of CO_2 that is exhaled by controlling the speed and depth of breathing in reaction to the blood CO_2 levels (as the primary driver for respiratory rate). The volume of CO_2 exhaled, and consequently the pH of the blood, increases as breathing becomes faster and deeper. By adjusting the speed and depth of breathing, the brain and lungs are able to regulate the blood pH to some degree in a reasonably quick manner. This is known as respiratory control of the acid/base balance.[12,15]

METABOLIC CONTROL OF THE ACID/BASE BALANCE

The kidneys are also able to regulate blood pH, and have a powerful effect by excreting excess acids or bases as required, as well as reabsorbing and regenerating bicarbonate. The kidneys can alter the amount of acid or base that is excreted dependent upon the body's needs, but because the kidneys make these adjustments more slowly, this compensation generally takes several days.

The kidney is the chief acid excretory system in the body and actively excretes H^+ ions from the proximal and distal tubules and the collecting duct of the nephrons. Overall, this removes acids from the body. The H^+ ions are lost in urine as water, ammonium, and sodium dihydrogen phosphate (see Figure 4.6). The kidneys also provide two major mechanisms for controlling bicarbonate. HCO_3^- reclamation occurs in the proximal tubule, where 90% of it is reabsorbed, and HCO_3^- regeneration occurs in the distal tubule and collecting ducts.[27]

When an H^+ ion is secreted into the ultrafiltrate in the nephron tubule, a Na^+ ion is simultaneously exchanged. This is an active process using adenosine triphosphate, and is important as it rids the body of excess acid, helps maintain pH, maintains ionic equivalence, conserves sodium, and also regenerates sodium bicarbonate for buffering. Once

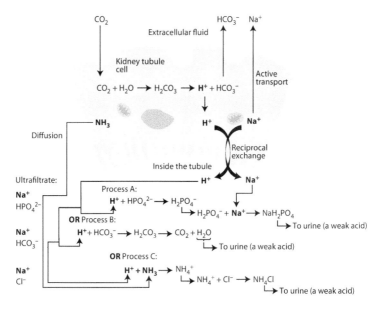

Figure 5.2 Renal excretion and transport of H^+.

in the ultrafiltrate, the transport of H^+ ions tends to occur by one of three methods.[12,15,27] H^+ ions may bind with bicarbonate to form carbonic acid and then break down into CO_2 and H_2O in the ultrafiltrate. Alternatively, ammonia (NH_3) may be utilized as a vehicle for losing H^+ ions. NH_3 reacts with an H^+ ion in the form ammonium (NH_4) in the ultrafiltrate, combining with Cl^- ions to form NH_4Cl. Lastly, the phosphate buffer system may come into play, in which hydrogen phosphate (HPO_4^{2-}) in the ultrafiltrate acts as an H^+ acceptor, forming $H_2PO_4^-$ (see Figure 5.2).[15,73]

Figure 5.3 demonstrates a comparison of the speeds of the various mechanisms in the body for the control of pH.

IMBALANCE

Acidosis and alkalosis are the two types of abnormality occurring in the acid/base balance. With acidosis, there is an excess of acid or too little base in the blood, resulting in a decrease in blood pH. With alkalosis, the blood has too much base, or too little acid, resulting in an increase in pH.

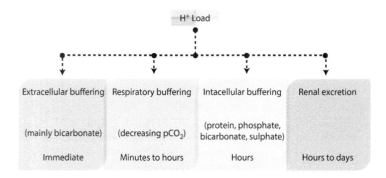

Figure 5.3 Response rates of control systems.

Acidosis and alkalosis may result from a wide variety of acute or chronic disorders, and can be categorized as metabolic or respiratory, depending on their primary cause. For example, acid accumulation in the blood caused by acute respiratory failure and insufficient clearance of CO_2 is known as an acute respiratory acidosis, whereas an excess loss of HCl due to vomiting would cause an acute metabolic alkalosis. See Table 5.1 for a summary of the most common causes of acid/base imbalance.

✗ CLINICAL FOCUS

Vomiting and diarrhea can cause acid/base and electrolyte abnormalities. Considering the composition of the normal stool is useful for understanding the consequences of diarrhea (see Chapter 2). The normal stool is alkaline, and for acid/base and electrolyte abnormalities to occur in diarrhea, the volume of fluid lost must be sufficiently large to overcome the kidney's ability to maintain acid/base equilibrium. When losses are sufficiently large, the disorder that develops is determined by the specific electrolyte content of the losses. Generally, severe diarrheal states can result in metabolic alkalosis with increased losses of H+ ions. Likewise, severe losses of gastro-intestinal fluids through vomiting also result in metabolic alkalosis.[75]

Acidosis and alkalosis are also categorized as compensated, partially compensated, or uncompensated, reflecting the degree to which the body has managed to maintain homeostasis with its regulatory mechanisms. For a primarily respiratory disorder, compensation is achieved

Table 5.1 Common causes of acidosis and alkalosis

Disorder	pH	H+	Causes
Metabolic acidosis	↓	↑	Renal failure, shock, infection, uncontrolled diabetes mellitus, lactic acidosis, starvation, and severe gastro-intestinal disturbance
Metabolic alkalosis	↑	↓	Usually from excessive HCl losses with vomiting/suction or renal losses with diuretics; rarely from excessive HCO_3 administration
Respiratory acidosis	↓	↑	Acute and chronic respiratory disease, hypoventilation, narcotics, anesthetics, or barbiturates
Respiratory alkalosis	↑	↓	Hyperventilation with altitude, anxiety, infection, asthma, embolism, drug overdose, carbon monoxide poisoning, or response to metabolic acidosis

through the excretion of acids or bases by the kidney, whilst for a primarily metabolic disorder, compensation will occur through the excretion or retention of CO_2 through respiration.[12,15,73] For example, if the patient has a metabolic acidosis, a compensatory mechanism would be to increase the respiratory rate to remove additional CO_2. If a patient has a metabolic alkalosis, the compensatory mechanism would be for the respiratory rate to decrease in order to increase blood CO_2. Table 5.2 reflects the changes that occur with acidosis and alkalosis and the body's compensatory responses in terms of serum bicarbonate levels and arterial pressure of CO_2 ($PaCO_2$; usually measured in mmHg).

✖ CLINICAL FOCUS

READING ARTERIAL BLOOD GASES

An arterial blood gas sample is obtained by sampling arterial blood. This is an advanced skill and not normally performed by students or novice practitioners. The most common site that is used is the radial artery; the femoral artery site may be used (especially if blood pressure is low in critically ill patients, when the radial pulse might be difficult to find). The arterial blood is then analyzed rapidly and a printout of the results is generated (such as in Figure 5.4).

```
PH_____7.490
PCO2_____42.3 mmHg
PO2_____88 mmHg
HCO3_____32 mmol/L
BEecf_____9 mmol/L
sO2*_____97 %
     *calculated


FIO2_____: 21
Sample Type_: ART

   24MAY01     11:25
```

Figure 5.4 Arterial blood gas results printout.

The order of the six blood gas values that are normally given in a report is pH, $PaCO_2$, PaO_2, HCO_3, BEecf, and SaO_2.

- pH = arterial blood pH
- $PaCO_2$ (or PCO_2) = arterial pressure of CO_2 in mmHg
- PaO_2 (or PO_2) = arterial pressure of O_2 in mmHg
- HCO_3 = serum bicarbonate concentration in mEq/L or mmol/L
- BEecf = base excess (extracellular fluid)
- SaO_2 saturation = percentage of Hb saturated with O_2 (also known as SO_2)

- FiO_2 = fraction of inhaled gas that is O_2 (normally 21%) is also usually given

Bicarbonate is sometimes referred to as standard bicarbonate and is calculated in order to help disregard respiratory status. Base excess indicates the required amount of base/acid needed to correct any pH imbalance. If positive, the patient has excess base (is alkalotic); if negative, the patient has insufficient base (is acidotic). Biochemistry such as serum potassium may also be given.

Table 5.2 Responses to acidosis and alkalosis

Disorder	pH	H+	Primary disturbance	Body's response
Metabolic acidosis	↓	↑	Decreased HCO_3	Increase respiratory rate
Metabolic alkalosis	↑	↓	Increased HCO_3	Decrease respiratory rate
Respiratory acidosis	↓	↑	Increased $PaCO_2$	Buffer with HCO_3
Respiratory alkalosis	↑	↓	Decreased $PaCO_2$	Reduce serum HCO_3

$PaCO_2$

$PaCO_2$ reflects *ventilation* and is the term that is used to describe the movement of gases into and out of the lungs. We can assess how well a person is ventilating by measuring $PaCO_2$. Abnormalities of ventilation will result in either an elevated $PaCO_2$ or a decreased $PaCO_2$. Hypoventilation is the term that is used to describe inadequate ventilation (i.e., a $PaCO_2$ >45 mmHg), whilst hyperventilation is the term that is used to describe excess ventilation (i.e., a $PaCO_2$ <35 mmHg). Hypoventilation will result in acid retention and one would expect a matching lowered pH (i.e., high $PaCO_2$ and low pH). Overall, we know what processes produce $PaCO_2$ as a byproduct of metabolism (and consume O_2). We know a person is adequately moving gases into and out of their lungs (ventilating) if the $PaCO_2$ is in the normal range (35–45 mmHg). If the $PaCO_2$ is normal, it is unlikely that the primary problem is respiratory.

HCO_3^-

HCO_3^- represents the available serum bicarbonate and reflects renal metabolic activity. With metabolic acidosis, excess acid (either by the addition of acid or the loss of bicarbonate) results in a low pH and low HCO_3^-. With metabolic alkalosis, excess bicarbonate (either from the addition of alkali or the loss of acid) results in a high pH and elevated HCO_3^-. Why does the concentration of HCO_3^- become low with the addition of acid? When acid is added, bicarbonate will bind the excess acid in order to buffer and neutralize it; hence, the concentration of free HCO_3^- declines. In respiratory disorders, HCO_3^- remains relatively unchanged initially.[73]

COMPENSATION

Compensation reflects the degree to which the body has managed to maintain homeostasis with its regulatory mechanisms. For a primary respiratory disorder, compensation is achieved by the excretion of acids or bases by the kidneys. For a primary metabolic disorder, compensation is achieved by the excretion or retention $PaCO_2$ through respiration.[15,73]

INTERPRETING ARTERIAL BLOOD GAS RESULTS

In examining a patient's arterial blood gas results, undertake the following steps:

1. Examine pH. Is it high (alkalosis) or low (acidosis)? Determine which.
2. Examine $PaCO_2$. Determine the patient's ventilation status and compare it with the pH.
   Is the pH low (acid) and the $PaCO_2$ high?
   - If YES, the person likely has a respiratory acidosis.
   - If NO, the person likely has a metabolic acidosis.
   Is the pH high (alkali) and the $PaCO_2$ low?
   - If YES, the person likely has a respiratory alkalosis.
   - If NO, the person likely has a metabolic alkalosis.
3. Examine HCO_3^-. Determine metabolic status and compare it with the pH.
   Is the pH low (acid) and the HCO_3^- low?
   - If YES, the person likely has a metabolic acidosis.
   Is the pH high (alkali) and the HCO_3^- normal or elevated?
   - If YES, the person likely has a metabolic alkalosis.
4. Determine if any compensation exists. Are there any mechanisms for compensation for acidosis or alkalosis?
   Is partial or complete compensation evident?
   a. Total compensation:
      i. pH normal
      ii. Possibly a prior problem
   b. Partial compensation (usually chronic):
      i. pH abnormal
      ii. HCO_3^- and $PaCO_2$ both abnormal

c. Uncompensated (usually acute):
   i. pH abnormal
   ii. HCO_3^- or $PaCO_2$ abnormal

CASE EXAMPLES

1. Mr. Smith is a 54-year-old man with a history of cardio-pulmonary disease. He had smoked a pack of cigarettes a day for more than 20 years, but had given up smoking 3 years ago. He has been taking erythromycin 500 mg 4 times a day (QID) for 3 days for an upper respiratory tract infection, and also has salbutamol inhalers prescribed. This afternoon, he was complaining of an acute shortness of breath and had the following vital signs: blood pressure (BP) 170/105; heart rate (HR) 85; respiratory rate (RR) 21; temperature (T) 37. His breath sounds are diminished to the lung bases with some fine crackles audible; O_2 saturation: 92% on room air. Arterial blood gases have been taken and have returned the following results:

- pH 7.18
- $PaCO_2$ 66
- PaO_2 55
- HCO_3^- 24
- SaO_2 92%

How can we explain these values?

  1. His pH is low (acid). 2. His $PaCO_2$ is high. 3. His HCO_3^- is normal.

  The match between his high $PaCO_2$ and pH suggests a respiratory acidosis, and he has a problem with hypoventilation. This is also supported by the rather low SaO_2 and PaO_2 values. Currently, this is uncompensated, as his HCO_3^- is normal, although at the lower limit.

2. Ms. Bush is a 28-year-old college student who has had type I diabetes mellitus since the age of 7 years. She recently developed influenza-like symptoms and went to see her family general practitioner after a week. The general practitioner subsequently referred her to the hospital. On admission, she had the following vital signs: BP 110/60; HR 86; RR 24, and blood was taken for biochemistry. The results were: glucose 15.4 mmol/L, Na^+ 131 mmol/L, Cl^- 80 mmol/L, K^+ 5.8 mmol/L.

Arterial blood gases were also taken and returned the following results:

- pH 7.18
- $PaCO_2$ 22
- PaO_2 82
- HCO_3^- 10
- SaO_2 98%

How can we explain these values?

1. Her pH is low (acid). 2. Her $PaCO_2$ is low. 3. $PaCO_2$ and SaO_2 are both normal (ventilation appears adequate). 4. Her HCO_3^- is low.

The match between her low HCO_3^- and pH suggests a metabolic acidosis. She likely has a problem with her serum bicarbonate due to diabetic ketoacidosis. Both her $PaCO_2$ and HCO_3^- are abnormal, so there is some partial compensation. Buffering is using up these resources in the body faster than they can be replaced.

🌐 TRIVIA

Pulse oximeters have become widespread in many clinical areas today. Can a pulse oximeter give you the same information as the PaO_2 from an arterial blood gas? The answer is no; the pulse oximeter does not measure the same thing as an arterial blood gas. The pulse oximeter measures the Hb oxygen saturation, while the arterial blood gas measures the pressure of oxygen gas dissolved in the blood (oxygen not bound to Hb).

Changes associated with different stages of the lifespan

6

SPECIFIC LEARNING OUTCOMES

By the end of this section, you will be able to:

- Describe the general changes in fluid and electrolyte physiology across the lifespan
- Compare and contrast the fluid and electrolyte requirements in preterm babies, neonates, infants, children, adults, and older adults
- Outline the three major buffering systems in the body

DEVELOPMENTAL CHANGES

Fluid composition remains relatively constant in the body throughout the developmental stages, although the total body water changes throughout human development and also varies with body weight and sex (see Table 6.1). These differences can generally be explained through differences in body fat, which is essentially water free.[76] Infants and young children have a greater water content than adults. For example, fluid constitutes approximately 75%–80% of the body weight in full-term infants. In adult men, body water accounts for approximately 60% of the body weight during adulthood and decreases to approximately 55% in older adults. In young women, it is approximately 52%, and in elderly women, approximately 46%.

As fluid volume changes throughout human development, disorders affecting the fluid status of infants, children, and older adults are particularly serious. Obesity produces further decreases in body water, sometimes reducing these levels to values as low as 30%–40% of the body weight in adults.[15]

Table 6.1 Body fluid variations by age and sex (References 8 and 76)

Age	Fluid percentage of total body weight
Prenatal (premature)	85%
Neonate	70%–80%
Child (1–12 years)	64%
Adult	Male: 60%
	Female: 52%
Older adult (>60 years)	Male: 55%
	Female: 46%

PRETERM INFANTS

The fluid requirements of premature infants vary considerably depending on gestational age and birth weight. Compared with full-term infants, premature infants have increased total fluid needs caused by greater insensible water losses through immature skin and exacerbated by the larger surface area-to-body weight ratio.

✖ CLINICAL FOCUS

A very premature infant may have a birth weight of less than 1000 g and may require between 120 and 220 mL/kg/day of water in order to maintain normal fluid and electrolyte balance.[77] As the degree of prematurity increases, the ability of various organs to carry out their normal functions is limited. The premature kidney is less able to concentrate urine effectively or to reabsorb sodium and bicarbonate. Therefore, the specific gravity of urine may be lower than normal.

NEONATES

Infants that are less than a month old have physical proportions and body compositions that are quite different from those of adults. Approximately 75% of the weight of a term infant is fluid, and their fluid and electrolyte requirements differ considerably from those of adults and older children, although their electrolyte biochemistry is not significantly different. Both the infant's body weight and age after delivery can be used as guides to calculating the total amount of fluid that is required daily. Fluid requirements increase slightly from birth to day 5 and then stabilize. For the first few days after delivery, the kidneys of the newborn infant produce little urine. The infant also has sufficient stores of extracellular fluid (ECF) at birth to maintain homeostasis over this period and, as a result, the infant does not need a lot of fluid in the first few days of life. The mother's milk production is also limited at this time. However, the infant's fluid needs gradually increase as renal function becomes established. By day 5, a lot more urine is passed and therefore fluid requirements increase.

Neonates need more fluid per kilogram than adults because they lose more fluid through their thinner skin as insensible water loss. They also lose more fluid from their lungs with their rapid respiratory rate, and their immature kidneys do not concentrate urine very well at this stage. They generally require:

- Day 1: 60 mL/kg
- Day 2: 75 mL/kg
- Day 3: 100 mL/kg
- Day 4: 125 mL/kg
- Day 5 (and thereafter): 150 mL/kg

Electrolytes obtained from the infant during the first day of life tend to reflect the values of the mother pre-delivery, and are not normally significantly different from adult values.[15,77]

CLINICAL FOCUS

- Neonatal jaundice or hyperbilirubinemia is the yellowing of the skin and other tissues in the newborn infant. A bilirubin level of more than 5 mg/dL indicates neonatal jaundice. This is caused by an excess of bilirubin in the blood that has not been taken up by the immature liver and not excreted effectively by the immature kidneys. This condition is common, being present in upwards of 70% of newborns.[78] It usually resolves spontaneously, but may be treated in the hospital with phototherapy in order to avoid bilirubin toxicity affecting the central nervous system. Exposing the neonate to specific light wavelengths (usually blue light) helps break down bilirubin in the skin. This treatment tends to increase insensible water loss and fluid requirements.

> ■ Diabetes insipidus is also a condition that is often diagnosed in neonates, being characterized by the excretion of large amounts of dilute urine due to an ADH deficiency or an insensitivity of the kidneys to ADH's effects. This results in an inability of the kidneys to concentrate urine and considerable fluid loss, with the typical symptoms of thirst. Diabetes insipidus is rare, affecting 1 in 25,000 people, with males and females equally affected.[79]

INFANTS

Infants (1 month to 1 year old) also have physical proportions and body compositions that are quite different from those of adults and are very susceptible to changes in their fluid and electrolyte balance. They have a higher metabolic rate, larger percentage of ECF, and greater body surface area compared to older children and adults. The total body water of an infant decreases from approximately 75%–80% at birth to approximately 67% at the end of the first year of life. At birth, the infant's ECF is greater than the intracellular fluid (ICF), and approximately half of an infant's ECF is exchanged daily.[77] The infant's anterior fontanel usually closes by 18 months of age, but in the young infant, the fontanel appears flat, often with visible pulsations, and can be an indicator of hydration status, as it appears sunken when the infant is dehydrated. Infants will normally urinate at least six times during the day and may have several soft, formed stools with higher water content than in the adult. Normal water losses occur through the kidneys, gastro-intestinal tract, skin, and respiratory tract in the normal way, and must be replaced. In general, infants weighing less than 10 kg require 100 mL/kg of fluid daily, whilst

✖ CLINICAL FOCUS

A common and serious cause of fluid and electrolyte problems in infants is gastroenteritis. This is an inflammation of the gastro-intestinal tract and is most commonly caused by viral infection, with rotavirus being a major cause. Other viruses that are known to cause gastroenteritis in infants include retrovirus, coxsackievirus, adenovirus, parvovirus, and poliovirus. Bacterial or parasitic cases of gastroenteritis also occur, although less frequently in infants.[81]

The fecal–oral route is the normal route of infection and the incubation period is normally between 24 and 48 hours. Affected infants experience vomiting, diarrhea, fever, abdominal pain, and weight loss. Fever often accompanies gastroenteritis and causes an increased insensible water loss through the skin and also in the lungs due to an increased respiratory rate. These symptoms predispose the infant to fluid and electrolyte loss, and potassium and chloride losses may be significant. An electrolyte imbalance may result, with metabolic alkalosis occurring due to prolonged vomiting and loss of hydrochloric acid. The infant can become dehydrated rapidly and careful rehydration therapy with appropriate electrolyte replacement is the normal treatment.

infants above 10 kg require 1000 mL plus 50 mL/kg weight over 10 kg. For example, an infant weighing 13 kg requires 1150 mL of fluid daily.[80]

CHILDREN

Children (1–12 years of age) have physical proportions that differ from those found in adults. They have a higher metabolic rate, a slightly greater percentage of ECF, and a greater body surface area compared to adults.[15] Approximately 64% of the weight of a child is fluid, and their electrolyte requirements are generally similar to those of adults, but differ in terms of the volumes required relative to their size, and those needed to support growth and development. Fluid requirements in children are calculated based on body weight according to the Holliday–Segar method.[80] Fluid requirements are better estimated by weight than age in order to account for the possibility of an underweight or overweight child.[80] Children above 10 kg require 1000 mL plus 50 mL/kg for each kilogram over 10 kg, whilst those over 20 kg need 1500 mL plus 20 mL/kg for each kilogram over 20 kg (see Table 6.2).

Table 6.2 Holliday–Segar fluid requirement calculation

Body weight	Fluid required
1–10 kg	100 mL/kg
10–20 kg	1000 mL plus 50 mL/kg for each kilogram over 10 kg
>20 kg	1500 mL plus 20 mL/kg for each kilogram over 20 kg

✕ CLINICAL FOCUS

Children between 12 and 36 months of age are commonly referred to as toddlers and as this is a key exploratory developmental stage, they are mainly at risk of fluid and electrolyte imbalances through injuries and infections. Burns and gastroenteritis are particularly problematic here. Less frequently, congenital kidney disease may also become apparent at this age.[81]

Burns are injuries that may be caused by heat, cold, electricity, chemicals, light, radiation, or friction. Tissue damage to the skin and underlying structures results. Any burn affecting more than 1% of the child's body surface (approximately the area of the child's palm) should be referred for medical attention. Burns may be classified as of superficial thickness (first-degree with epidermis involvement), of partial thickness (second-degree with dermis damage), and of full thickness (third-degree with dermis and underlying tissue damage). Fluid and electrolyte loss is considerably increased in areas where the skin has been damaged with burns through insensible loss and loss of interstitial fluid. For this reason, estimation of the body surface area (BSA) damage is important in estimating the child's fluid needs. In children and infants, the Lund–Browder method is often used to assess the burned BSA, as the combined surface area of the head and neck to the surface area of the limbs is typically larger in children than in adults. This method attributes different percentages of BSA to different parts of the body. For example, the anterior head of a child is estimated at 4.5% BSA in the adult and 8.5% BSA in a child.[82]

The most important aspect of early care of the burned child is the initiation of the volume replacement of large quantities of isotonic fluids that are sufficient to maintain organ perfusion. Because of the greater variability between BSA and weight in a child than in an adult, an accurate estimation of the resuscitation requirements is best based on BSA, as determined from nomograms of height and weight. For children, initial resuscitation is usually based on 5000 mL/m^2 BSA burned per day plus 2000 mL/m^2 BSA total/day of fluid.[83]

ADOLESCENTS

The fluid and electrolyte physiology of adolescents is not significantly different from that of adults. However, the accelerated growth during adolescence requires additional nutritional support, including adequate fluids and minerals.

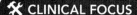

CLINICAL FOCUS

As adolescence is the time when identity and emotional independence develops more, the physical, emotional, and social changes can make some behavioral fluid- and electrolyte-related problems apparent. Adolescents often experiment with recreational drugs (including alcohol), which may lead to acute episodes of dehydration, such as using methylenedioxymethamphetamine or "ecstasy", which raises body temperature.[84] Eating disorders such as anorexia nervosa and bulimia can also influence electrolyte balance.[85]

Anorexia nervosa involves the inability to maintain a minimally normal body weight and the occurrence of severe weight loss in the absence of physical causes.[85] It is a complex eating disorder involving a preoccupation with food, weight, and body image, resulting in persistent dieting in order to lose weight, which can lead to severe malnutrition. The incidence is approximately 7% of the total population, so it is a significant disorder. It occurs primarily in female adolescents (only approximately 5% of cases are in men). It has a mortality rate of approximately 4%, with the major risk factor being an admission body mass index below 15 kg/m^2.[86] If untreated, anorexia can progress to serious fluid and electrolyte imbalances due to insufficient dietary intake (especially hypophosphatemia), which leads to hypotension and cardiac dysrhythmias. Bone loss, osteoporosis, and renal disease are also comorbidities that can occur. Treatment is primarily behaviorally focused, but also often includes medical treatment.[87]

ADULTS

As we have seen, the physical proportions and body compositions of adults result in fluids accounting for approximately 60% of body weight in men and approximately 52% of body weight in women. Therefore, any disorders that upset the fluid and electrolyte balance will have significant effects upon individuals.

FLUID AND ELECTROLYTE CHANGES IN PREGNANCY

For pregnant women, fluid and electrolyte needs increase significantly to meet the needs of the growing fetus. As the placenta and fetus develop, blood flow to the uterus must increase to approximately 1 L/minute (20%

of normal cardiac output) by term in order to meet the demands of the utero-placental circulation. The volume of the utero-placental circulation increases markedly. Progesterone and aldosterone production increases during pregnancy, leading to an expansion of the maternal plasma volume by approximately 40%. Therefore, hematocrit decreases slightly, and fluid may account for up to 6 lbs of weight in the ECF compartment. This additional sodium and fluid will be excreted postpartum.[15,88]

The additional ECF and volume increase predispose pregnant women to dependent edema during the later pregnancy, and more generalized edema can also occur; overall, approximately three-quarters of pregnant women experience edema at some stage during pregnancy. Although body sodium is retained during pregnancy, an increase in ADH also causes H_2O retention, and the increased ECF maintains a normal or slightly lowered plasma sodium level. Osmolality may actually decrease by 10 mmol/kg. Likewise, potassium is retained during pregnancy to meet the fetal growth needs, but serum potassium levels decrease slightly due to the volume dilution of the ECF. Magnesium levels are normally slightly lower during pregnancy as the fetal demands make an impact on maternal magnesium stores. Calcium needs increase significantly during pregnancy, and serum calcium is lowered, particularly in the second or third trimester. This can be aggravated by the lowered serum albumin (a calcium binding protein) level. However, the calcium needs can normally be met by regular dietary intake, as parathyroid hormone increases calcium absorption in the gut. After birth and during lactation, the mother's calcium needs will increase to meet the demands of the growing baby. Serum phosphate levels remain normal during pregnancy.[88] Metabolic alkalosis can develop with hyperemesis in early pregnancy, and progesterone has a stimulating effect on the respiratory center in the brain and may cause hyperventilation and the arterial pressure of carbon dioxide to decrease, causing mild respiratory alkalosis. Therefore, in late pregnancy, it may the normal to have slightly lowered serum bicarbonate.[88]

✖ CLINICAL FOCUS

Diabetes mellitus is a key example of a metabolic disorder having a significant impact on fluid balance. It is a chronic disease that is associated with abnormally high levels of glucose in the blood. Diabetes mellitus results from one of two mechanisms: either inadequate production of insulin or inadequate sensitivity of cells to the action of insulin. In both cases, glucose cannot easily move from the ECF into the ICF, so blood glucose levels are elevated. Although it can occur in all age groups, it is relatively common in young adults (18–30 years of age). Some of the excess glucose in the blood is filtered into the ultrafiltrate by the kidneys as the renal threshold for glucose is reached. This results in a reduced reabsorption of water from the nephron tubules and collecting ducts, causing significant diuresis (polyuria) and excessive thirst (polydipsia).

With an increase in the catabolism of fat to meet the body's energy requirements, diabetic ketoacidosis may result due to the increased production of acidic ketone bodies by the liver. The ketone bodies increase the osmolarity of the blood and are acidic. Diabetic ketoacidosis can become severe enough to result in unconsciousness from the combination of metabolic acidosis and hypovolemic shock with dehydration.[58,89] Alternatively, hyperosmolar non-ketoacidotic coma may occur in diabetes mellitus, where hyperglycemia and dehydration alone are sufficient to cause unconsciousness.

Dehydration in adults is rare from deficient oral intake, but may also result from fever or exposure to hot and arid environments without adequate rehydration. In both of these cases, dehydration results from an increased insensible loss of water from the skin and lungs. Dehydration and exposure in hot environments may also lead to the complication of heat stroke, which is also more common in adults due to their exposure to the environment. Heat stroke may arise when long, extreme exposure to the sun occurs and the individual is unable to sweat enough to lower their body temperature. Loss of consciousness and seizures may result. Dehydration and electrolyte imbalances in adults may also occur through prolonged gastroenteritis.

Acute renal failure is another major cause of fluid and electrolyte imbalance seen in adults. It is a common complication of critical illness, occurring in anywhere from 1% to 25% of critically ill patients and significantly increases the risk of mortality.[90] Acute damage to the renal nephrons occurs as a result of trauma, toxicity, acute disease processes, or, more commonly, impaired renal perfusion. Although deaths from acute renal failure are decreasing, the incidence of the condition is increasing, from 61 cases per 100,000 of the population in 1988 to 288 cases per 100,000 of the population in 2002. The reasons for this are unclear, but increases in sepsis and an older population have been discussed as possible factors.[91]

If untreated, acute tubular necrosis usually results and nephron tubules become permanently damaged. Initial damage may result in nephrotic syndrome, a non-specific disorder in which the nephrons become more porous and reabsorption is impaired, causing them to leak large amounts of protein and fluid (proteinuria) into the urine. In all cases of acute renal failure, fluid retention, electrolyte imbalance (particularly hyperkalemia), and acidosis are severe problems requiring hospital treatment.

OLDER ADULTS

In the older adult (60 years of age and above), the percentage of body fluid weight drops slightly by approximately 5%. This is mainly due to changes in body weight distribution, with a decrease in muscle mass relative to fat in the body. A variety of conditions are more common in this age group, but as previously noted, these conditions are not restricted to these age groups.[15]

✖ CLINICAL FOCUS

- Hyponatremia is a condition in which plasma Na^+ falls below 135 mmol/L (see Tables 3.2 and 3.3 and Figure 3.1) and has been cited as the most common electrolyte disorder in North America, with increasing incidence among hospitalized and nursing home patients.[92] One common cause of hyponatremia in older adults is that which is associated with diuretic use for cardiovascular conditions. Many diuretics (e.g., furosemide) increase Na^+ loss as a side effect. Hyperosmolar hypernatremia may also result when there is considerable loss of Na^+ and fluid replacement by inappropriately hypotonic fluids (such as tap water). This may result from vomiting, diarrhea, excess sweating, or burns. Hyponatremia is normally asymptomatic, but hyperosmolar hyponatremia may cause cerebral edema with an osmotic shift of water from the plasma into the brain ICF, and typical symptoms would include nausea, vomiting, headache, and malaise. Treatment is by electrolyte replacement.
- Hypocalcemia is another clinical electrolyte imbalance that is frequently seen in older adults, particularly as a result of reduced

mobility, decreased calcium absorption with vitamin D deficiency, menopause, and decreased stomach acid in old age. The North American intake guidelines recommend that the adequate intake of vitamin D for people aged 51–70 years is 400 IU, and is 600 IU for people older than 70 years of age. In the older adult, it is thought diet alone seldom meets the adequate intake for calcium and vitamin D. In one well-publicized 2002 study of elderly people living in long-term care facilities, only one patient had achieved the adequate intake from dietary sources alone.[93] Most calcium is used for the development and maintenance of teeth and bones, and so chronic deficiency may result in weakness of these tissues in the older person.[15]

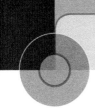

Glossary of key terms

Absorption: to move a substance into the body, such as the absorption of nutrients in the gastro-intestinal tract.

Acid: a substance that yields hydrogen ions when dissolved in water.

Atom: the smallest unit of an element that retains its chemical properties.

Atomic Weight: the average mass of an atom of an element, usually expressed relative to the mass of carbon-12, which is assigned 12 atomic mass units (symbol=amu). See also, Dalton.

Base: a substance that yields hydroxyl ions when dissolved in water, and reacts with acids to form salts.

Colloid: colloid-based (gelatinous) solutions.

Crystalloid: mineral-based solutions.

Dalton: a measure of atomic mass (symbol=Da, although amu is more commonly used today). Named after the English chemist John Dalton (1766–1844). One hydrogen atom has mass of 1 Da. A useful measure for the comparison of relative molecular mass (e.g., urea=60 Da, whilst albumin=68,000 Da). See also, Atomic Weight.

Diuresis: the excretion of an unusually large quantity of urine.

Divalent: having a valency of two; also known as bivalent.

Dry Weight: the lowest weight a patient can tolerate without the development of symptoms or hypotension. It is a term that is often used in nephrology with respect to dialysis.

Edema: an abnormal accumulation of fluid in the tissues of the body, causing swelling (from the Greek *oidēma* meaning swelling).

Electrolyte: a molecule that in solution separates into its ionic components and is capable of conducting electricity.

Euvolemic: not dehydrated or fluid overloaded.

Hematocrit: Ht or HCT, also known as packed cell volume (PCV) and erythrocyte volume fraction (EVF), it is the percentage of erythrocytes in blood. It is normally approximately 45% for men and approximately 40% for women.

Hypercalcemia: an abnormally high level of calcium in the blood.

Hyperkalemia: an abnormally high level of potassium in the blood.

Hypernatremia: an abnormally high level of sodium in the blood.

Hypertonic: having a higher osmotic pressure in a fluid compared to another fluid.

Hypocalcaemia: an abnormally low level of calcium in the blood.

Hypokalemia: an abnormally low level of potassium in the blood.

Hyponatremia: an abnormally low level of sodium in the blood.

Hypotonic: having a lesser osmotic pressure in a fluid compared to another fluid.

Ion: a positively or negatively charged particle.

Isotonic: having the same osmotic pressure in a fluid compared to another fluid.

Matter: anything that has mass.

Mole: symbol=mol. It is the unit that is used to measure the amount of molecules, and is the amount of a substance represented by 6.02×10^{23} atoms, molecules, ions, or elementary units of it. It is relative to the number of atoms in 12 g of carbon-12. One mole of carbon-12 weighs 12 g and contains 6.02×10^{23} carbon atoms.

Molecule: the simplest unit of a substance that retains its chemical and physical properties, consisting of two or more atoms combined, which can react in a chemical process.

Normovolemic: a normal volume of blood in the body.

Osmolality: this measures the concentration of osmotically active particles per kilogram (mass) of the solvent, commonly expressed as mmol/kg.

Osmolar Gap: this is the difference between measured serum osmolality and calculated serum osmolarity, used as a diagnostic tool in helping differentiate the causes of an elevated anion gap in metabolic acidosis. The normal osmolar gap is 10–15 mmol/L H_2O. An elevated osmolar gap may be seen in poisoning with ethylene glycol or methanol, alcoholic and diabetic ketoacidosis, lactic acidosis, and also in chronic renal failure.

Osmolarity: this is the concentration of osmotically active particles in a solution per liter (volume) of it. It is commonly expressed in mmol/L.

Osmole: a unit of osmotic pressure equivalent to the amount of solute that dissociates in solution to form one mole (Avogadro's constant of particles; molecules and ions). Symbol=Osm. It is practically the same as a mole, but is used as an indicator of osmotic pressure rather than the amount of a substance.

Ultrafiltrate: the substances in solution that pass through an ultrafilter (a semi-permeable membrane through which the filtrate passes under pressure). An example would be the filtrate in the nephron tubules filtered by the glomeruli.

Urine: liquid waste produced by the kidneys and temporarily stored in the bladder; urine is an amber, transparent fluid.

Valency: the combining capacity of an atom or radical determined by the number of electrons that it would lose, add, or share when reacting with other atoms (also known as valence). For example, hydrogen's valency is one. In addition, it is the number of binding sites of an antibody or antigen.

References

1. Barnes J. 1987. *Early Greek Philosophy*. London, UK, Penguin: 125–127.
2. Blakemore C, Jennett S. 2001. *Humours. The Oxford Companion to the Body*. Oxford, UK, Oxford University Press: 321–325.
3. Turner R. 1871. Blood-letting. *The British Medical Journal*. 1(533): 283–291.
4. Rose BD, Post TW, Stokes J. 2016. *Clinical Physiology of Acid–Base and Electrolyte Disorders* (6th Ed.). New York, NY, USA, McGraw-Hill: 478–479.
5. Keyes JL. 2007. *Fluid, Electrolyte, and Acid–Base Regulation* (2nd Ed.). Toronto, ON, Canada, Jones & Bartlett Publishers: 3–9, 14–15, 38–55.
6. Das D. 2008. *Fundamantals of Biochemistry* (13th Ed.). Kolkata, India, Academic Publishers: 121, 619–621.
7. Erstad BL. 2003. Osmolarity and osmolality: Narrowing the terminology gap. *Pharmacotherapy*. 23(9): 1085–1086.
8. Agrò FE. 2013. *Body Fluid Management; From Physiology to Therapy*. New York, NY, USA, Springer.
9. Luby-Phelps K. 2000. Cytoarchitecture and physical properties of cytoplasm: Volume, viscosity, diffusion, intracellular surface area. *International Review of Cytology*. 192: 189–221.
10. Roos A, Boron W. 1981. Intracellular pH. *Physiology Reviews*. 61(2): 296–434.
11. Voeikov VL. 2005. Fundamental role of water in bioenergetics. In Beloussov LV, Voeikov VL, Martynyuk S (Eds.), *Biophotonics and Coherent Systems in Biology*. New York, NY, USA, Springer: 89–129.
12. Halperin ML, Goldstein MD, Kamel KS. 2010. *Fluid, Electrolyte and Acid–Base Physiology: A Problem-Based Approach*. New York, NY, USA, W.B. Saunders Co.
13. Lo SY, Li WC, Huang SH. 1999. Water clusters in life. *Medical Hypotheses*. 54(6): 948–953.
14. Timmins PA, Wall JC. 1977. Bone water. *Calcified Tissue Research*. 23(1): 1–5.
15. Silverthorn DU. 2016. *Human Physiology: An Integrated Approach* (7th Ed.). Harlow, UK, Pearson Education: 678–716.

16. Chowdhury AH, Lobo DN. 2011. Fluids and gastrointestinal function. *Current Opinion in Clinical Nutrition and Metabolic Care.* 14(5): 469–476.

17. Noback C, Strominger N, Demarest R, Ruggiero D. 2005. *The Human Nervous System.* Totowa, NJ, USA, Humana Press: 93–95.

18. Platt PN. 1983. Examination of synovial fluid. *Clinics in Rheumatic Diseases.* 9(1): 51–67.

19. Frisbie DD Cross MW, McIlwraith CW. 2006. A comparative study of articular cartilage thickness in the stifle of animal species used in human pre-clinical studies compared to articular cartilage thickness in the human knee. *Veterinary and Comparative Orthopaedics and Traumatology.* 19(3): 142–146.

20. Salt AN. 2007. Cochlear fluids homeostasis and its relevance to drug delivery to the inner ear. *Equilibrium Research.* 66: 206–207.

21. Snell RS, Lemp MA. 1998. *Clinical Anatomy of the Eye* (2nd Ed.). Malden, MA, USA, Blackwell Science: 120–125.

22. Brace RA. 1997 Physiology of amniotic fluid volume regulation. *Clinical Obstetrics & Gynecology.* 40: 280–282.

23. Borg F. 2003. What is osmosis? Explanation and understanding of a physical phenomenon. Jyväskylä University, Chydenius Institute, Karleby, Finland. Retrieved April 21, 2009 from: http://arxiv.org/abs/physics/0305011v1

24. Williams JS, Williams GH. 2003. 50th anniversary of aldosterone. *The Journal of Clinical Endocrinology & Metabolism.* 88(6): 2364–2372.

25. Cauliez B, Berthe MC, Lavoinne A. 2005. Brain natriuretic peptide: Physiological, biological and clinical aspects. *Annales de Biologie Clinique.* 63(1): 15–25.

26. Hale A, Hovey J. 2013. *Fluid, Electrolyte, and Acid–Base Imbalances: Content Review Plus Practice Questions.* New York, NY, USA, F.A. Davis.

27. Rose BD, Post TW. 2016. *Clinical Physiology of Acid–Base and Electrolyte Disorders* (5th Ed.). New York, NY, USA, McGraw-Hill.

28. Fukagawa M, Kurokawa K, Papadakis MA. 2007. Fluid & electrolyte disorders. In McPhee SJ, Papadakis MA, Tierney LM (Eds.), *Current Medical Diagnosis and Treatment.* New York, NY, USA, McGraw Hill: 120–156, 167–192.

29. Andropoulos DB. 2012. Pediatric normal laboratory values. In Gregory GA, Andropoulos DB (Eds.), *Gregory's Pediatric Anesthesia* (5th Ed.). New York, NY, USA, Blackwell Publishing Ltd: 1301–1314.

30. Takahashi H, Yoshika M, Komiyama Y, Nishimura M. 2011. The central mechanism underlying hypertension: A review of the roles of sodium ions, epithelial sodium channels, the renin–angiotensin–aldosterone system, oxidative stress and endogenous digitalis in the brain. *Hypertension Research*. 34(11): 1147–1160.

31. Lindner G, Funk GC, Schwarz C, Kneidinger N, Kaider A, Schneeweiss B, Kramer L, Druml W. 2007. Hypernatraemia in the critically ill is an independent risk factor for mortality. *American Journal of Kidney Diseases: The Official Journal of the National Kidney Foundation*. 50(6): 952–957.

32. Reynolds RM, Padfield PL, Seckl JR. 2006. Disorders of sodium balance. *British Medical Journal*. 332(7543): 702–705.

33. Gennari FJ. 2002. Disorders of potassium homeostasis; hypokalemia and hyperkalemia. *Critical Care Clinics of North America*. 18: 273–288.

34. Greenlee M, Wingo CS, McDonough AA, Youn JH, Kone BC. 2009. Narrative review: Evolving concepts in potassium homeostasis and hypokalemia. *Annals of Internal Medicine*. 150: 619–625.

35. Salem MM, Rosa RM, Batlle DC. 1991. Extrarenal potassium tolerance in chronic renal failure: Implications for the treatment of acute hyperkalaemia. *American Journal of Kidney Diseases*. 18(4): 421–440.

36. Elliott MJ, Ronksley PE, Clase CM, Ahmed SB, Hemmelgarn BR. 2010. Management of patients with acute hyperkalemia. *Canadian Medical Association Journal*. 182(15): 1631–1635.

37. Alfonzo A, Soar J, MacTier R et al. 2014. Treatment of Acute Hyperkalemia in Adults. The Renal Association. Retrieved April 26, 2016 from: http://www.renal.org/guidelines/joint-guidelines/treatment-of-acute-hyperkalaemia-in-adults#sthash.vXcD0IG3.QqdB4c5G.dpbs

38. Sterns RH, Rojas M, Bernstein P, Chennupati S. 2010. Ion-exchange resins for the treatment of hyperkalemia: Are they safe and effective? *Journal of the American Society of Nephrology*. 21(5): 733–735.

39. Federal Drug Administration. 2015. FDA approves new drug to treat hyperkalemia. Retrieved May 26, 2016 from: http://www.fda.gov/NewsEvents/Newsroom/PressAnnouncements/ucm468546.htm

40. Lavie CJ, Crocker EF, Key KJ, Ferguson TG. 1986. Marked hypochloremic metabolic alkalosis with severe compensatory hypoventilation. *Southern Medical Journal.* 79(10): 1296–1299.
41. Quarles LD. 2003. Extracellular calcium-sensing receptors in the parathyroid gland, kidney, and other tissues. *Current Opinions in Nephrology and Hypertension.* 12: 349–355.
42. Vincent JL. 2009. Relevance of albumin in modern critical care medicine. *Best Practice and Research in Clinical Anaesthesiology.* 23(2): 183–191.
43. Jafri L, Khan AH, Azeem S. 2014. Ionized calcium measurement in serum and plasma by ion selective electrodes: Comparison of measured and calculated parameters. *Indian Journal of Clinical Biochemistry.* 29(3): 327–332.
44. Cho KC. 2016. Electrolyte and acid-base disorders. In Papadakis MA, MacPhee SJ, Rabow MW (Eds), *Current Medical Diagnosis and Treatment.* New York, NY, USA, McGraw-Hill Education: 324–398.
45. Takeda E, Taketani Y, Sawada N, Sato T, Yamamoto H. 2004. The regulation and function of phosphate in the human body. *Biofactors.* 21(1–4): 345–355.
46. Berner YN, Shike M. 1988. Consequences of phosphate imbalance. *Annual Review of Nutrition.* 8: 121–148.
47. Johnson RJ, Feehally J, Floege J. 2014. *Comprehensive Clinical Nephrology* (5th Ed.). New York, NY, USA, Mosby Inc.
48. Lederer E. 2012. Hypophosphataemia. Retrieved December 11, 2012 from: http://emedicine.medscape.com/article/242280-overview
49. Rude RK. 2012. Magnesium. In Ross AC, Caballero B, Cousins RJ, Tucker KL, Ziegler TR (Eds.), *Modern Nutrition in Health and Disease* (11th Ed.). Baltimore, MA, USA, Lippincott Williams & Wilkins: 159–175.
50. Arnaud MJ. 2008. Update on the assessment of magnesium status. *British Journal of Nutrition.* 99(Suppl. 3): S24–S36.
51. Elin RJ. 2010. Assessment of magnesium status for diagnosis and therapy. *Magnesium Research.* 23(4): S194–S198.
52. Chaudhary DP, Sharma R, Bansal DD. 2010. Implications of magnesium deficiency in type 2 diabetes: A review. *Biological Trace Element Research.* 134: 119–129.
53. Chojkier M. 2005. Inhibition of albumin synthesis in chronic diseases: Molecular mechanisms. *Journal of Clinical Gastroenterology.* 39(4 Suppl. 2): S143–S146.

54. Eljaiek R, Dubois MJ. 2012. Hypoalbuminaemia in the first 24h of admission is associated with organ dysfunction in burned patients. *Burns*. 29(1): 113–118.

55. Vincent JL, Abraham E, Patrick K, Moore FA, Fink MP. 2016. *Textbook of Critical Care*. Toronto, ON, Canada, Elsevier Canada.

56. Petrucci RH, Herring FG, Madura JD, Bissonette C. 2016. *General Chemistry: Principles & Modern Applications* (11th Ed.). Upper Saddle River, NJ, USA, Pearson Education.

57. Turner N, Goldsmith D, Winearls C. 2015. *Oxford Textbook of Clinical Nephrology* (4th Ed.). Oxford, UK, Oxford University Press.

58. Hall JE, Guyton AC. 2006. *Textbook of Medical Physiology*. St Louis, MO, USA, Elsevier Saunders.

59. Carafoli E. 1991. Calcium pump of the plasma membrane. *Physiology Review*. 71(1): 129–153.

60. Jensen TP, Buckby LE, Empson RM. 2004. Expression of plasma membrane Ca^{2+} ATPase family members and associated synaptic proteins in acute and cultured organotypic hippocampal slices from rat. *Developmental Brain Research*. 152(2): 129–136.

61. Wright EM. 2001. Renal Na^+–glucose co-transporters. *American Journal of Physiology—Renal Physiology*. 280(1): F10–F18.

62. Boron WF. 2007. *Medical Physiology: A Cellular and Molecular Approach*. London, UK, Elsevier/Saunders: 791–793.

63. Frost P. 2015. Intravenous fluid therapy in adult inpatients. *British Medical Journal (Clinical Research Ed.)*. 350: g7620.

64. National Institute for Health and Care Excellence. 2013. Intravenous Fluid Therapy. Clinical Guideline CG174. Retrieved January 5, 2016 from: https://www.nice.org.uk/guidance/cg174/evidence/intravenous-fluid-therapy-in-adults-in-hospital-full-guideline-191667997

65. Martin GS. 2008. An Update on Intravenous Fluids. Retrieved December 14, 2012 from http://www.medscape.org/viewarticle/503138

66. Frost PJ, Wise MP. 2012. Early management of acutely ill ward patients. *British Medical Journal*. 345: 43–47.

67. Garrett BM, Ong P, Galdas P. 2016. *Pocket Clinical Reference for Nurses* (3rd Ed.). Oxford, UK, Clinical Publishing Services.

68. Perel P, Roberts I, Ker K. 2013. Colloids versus crystalloids for fluid resuscitation in critically ill patients. *Cochrane Database of Systematic Reviews*. 2: CD000567.

69. Klabundle RE. 2011. *Cardiovascular Physiology Concepts*. New York, NY, USA, Lippincott Williams & Wilkins.

70. Rector FC, Brenner BM. 2004. *Brenner & Rector's the Kidney* (7th Ed.). Philadelphia, PA, USA, Saunders: 212–256.

71. Curran P, Macintosh J. 1962. A model system for biological water transport. *Nature*. 193: 347–348.

72. Covington AK, Bates RG, Durst RA. 1985. Definitions of pH scales, standard reference values, measurement of pH, and related terminology. *Pure Applied Chemistry*. 57(3): 531–542.

73. Seifter JL. 2014. Integration of acid–base and electrolyte disorders. *New England Journal of Medicine*. 371: 1821–1831.

74. Phillips JR, Cadwallader DE. 1971. Behavior of erythrocytes in phosphate buffer systems. *Journal of Pharmaceutical Sciences*. 60(7): 1033–1035.

75. Gennari FJ, Weise WJ. 2008. Acid–base disturbances in gastrointestinal disease. *Clinical Journal of the American Society of Nephrology*. 3(6): 1861–1868.

76. Metheny NM. 2000. *Fluids and Electrolyte Balance: Nursing Considerations* (4th Ed.). Philadelphia, PA, USA, Lippencott: 915–920.

77. Friedman A. 2005. Pediatric hydration therapy: Historical review and a new approach. *Kidney International*. 67(1): 380–388.

78. Amato M, Inaebnit D. 1991. Clinical usefulness of high intensity green light phototherapy in the treatment of neonatal jaundice. *European Journal of Pediatrics*. 150(4): 274–276.

79. Larsen PR. 2003. *Williams Textbook of Endocrinology*. Philadelphia, PA, USA, Saunders: 290.

80. Holliday MA, Segar WE. 1957. The maintenance need for water in parenteral fluid therapy. *Pediatrics*. 19(5): 823–832.

81. Eliason BE, Lewan RB. 1998. Gastroenteritis in children: Principles of diagnosis and treatment. *American Family Physician*. 58: 1769–1770.

82. Watts AM, Tyler MP, Perry ME, Roberts AH, McGrouther DA. 2001. Burn depth and its histological measurement. *Burns*. 27(2): 154–160.

83. Sheridan RL. 2001. Comprehensive treatment of burns. *Current Problems in Surgery*. 38(9): 657–756.

84. Huizink AC, Ferdinand RF, van der Ende J, Verhulst FC. 2006. Symptoms of anxiety and depression in childhood and use of MDMA: Prospective, population based study. *British Medical Journal (Clinical Research Ed.)*. 332(7545): 825–828.

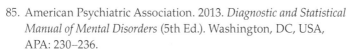

85. American Psychiatric Association. 2013. *Diagnostic and Statistical Manual of Mental Disorders* (5th Ed.). Washington, DC, USA, APA: 230–236.

86. Berkman ND, Lohr KN, Bulik CM. 2007. Outcomes of eating disorders: A systematic review of the literature. *International Journal of Eating Disorders*. 40(4): 293–309.

87. Bachrach LK, Guido D, Katzman D, Litt IF, Marcus R. 1990. Decreased bone density in adolescent girls with anorexia nervosa. *Pediatrics*. 86(3): 440–447.

88. Wylie L. 2010. *Essential Anatomy & Physiology in Maternity Care* (2nd Ed.). New York, NY, USA, Churchill Livingstone, Elsevier.

89. Paulson WD. 1986. Anion gap–bicarbonate relation in diabetic ketoacidosis. *American Journal of Medicine*. 105(6): 995–1000.

90. Bellomo R, Ronco C, Kellum JA, Mehta RL, Palevsky P. 2004. Acute renal failure—Definition, outcome measures, animal models, fluid therapy and information technology needs: The second international consensus conference of the Acute Dialysis Quality Initiative (ADQI) group. *Critical Care*. 8: R204–R212.

91. Xue JL, Daniels F, Star RA, Kimmel PL, Eggers PW, Molitoris BA, Himmelfarb J, Collins AJ. 2006. Incidence and mortality of acute renal failure in Medicare beneficiaries: 1992 to 2001. *Journal of the American Society of Nephrology*. 17: 1135–1142.

92. Upadhyay A, Jaber BL, Madias NE. 2006. Incidence and prevalence of hyponatraemia. *American Journal of Medicine*. 119(7 Suppl. 1): S30–S35.

93. Lee LT, Drake WM, Kendler DM. 2002. Intake of calcium and vitamin D in 3 Canadian long-term care facilities. *Journal of the American Dietetic Association*. 102(2): 244–247.

94. Stelfox HT, Ahmed SB, Khandwala F, Zygun D, Shahpori R, Laupland K. 2008. The epidemiology of intensive care unit-acquired hyponatraemia and hypernatraemia in medical–surgical intensive care units. *Critical Care*. 12(6): R162.

Index